AIDS
AND THE
HEALER
WITHIN

NICK BAMFORTH

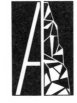

AMETHYST BOOKS
NEW YORK   LONDON

This book is dedicated to Denise Cooney and Tom Ruggiero for, each in their own way, kicking me in the right direction and to Tom Simpson, my sister June and the rest of my family and friends who have given me such support.

Published in the United States by
Amethyst Books, 160 West 71st Street,
Apt. 17D, New York, N.Y. 10023
and in the United Kingdom by
Amethyst Books, 44 Gledstanes Road,
London W14.

Designed by Paperweight

Library of Congress Catalog Card Number:
87-72727

ISBN 0–944256–00–7

Amethyst Books are distributed in the United
States by Publishers Group West, Emeryville,
Ca. and in the United Kingdom by
Gateway Books, Bath.

Contents

Introduction

This book is written for the thousands of people who either have AIDS or are afraid of coming down with the disease, as well as for those who care for people with AIDS.

Its aim is quite simply to teach how each and every one of us is able to assume total responsibility for our own health instead of passively relying on traditional medicine to find a cure for us. If you are convinced that AIDS, or for that matter any disease, is something over which you have no control, then this book is definitely not for you.

This book is broadly based on my Healer Within workshop, as well as the experience I have gained and the knowledge I have picked up from the many individual healing sessions I have done with people with AIDS.

Whenever I read a newspaper or listen to the latest words of doom from the medical profession, I sometimes wonder whether I live in the same world, for so many of the experiences that I have shared with people with AIDS, ARC (AIDS Related Complex) or who are antibody positive have been positive and filled with hope and love.

For there is hope, and in denying people hope, the press and the medical profession bear a heavy responsibility. In putting forward their own limited and negative understanding of AIDS as the only reality, they are taking away the one thing that enables someone to fight this disease: the strength within an individual.

Over the past few years, I have got to know many people who have discovered this inner strength through the challenge that AIDS has offered them. Those who have been diagnosed with AIDS and continue to remain relatively stable over a long period of time are quite simply those who have taken their lives into their own hands. Many have recognized that their lives before they got sick were by no means wonderful, and, in doing so, they have set out on a path towards discovering what is really important in their lives, what is really special within them.

This is also the path towards health and recovery. As the mind and spirit finds its own true strength, so does the body.

What I am going to ask you to do in reading this book is to start looking at your life in a new way – one in which you recognize not only that it is your right but also that it is within your power to create health and harmony in your life. And I do not mean this just in terms of ridding yourself of the disease we call AIDS; the potential of that creativity within us goes far beyond this to cover every aspect of our existence from relationships to prosperity in its broadest sense.

All of us at some point feel a yearning for something deeper within ourselves, something more meaningful than the day to day existence we lead. For so many people I know, myself included, AIDS has been the stimulus to recognize this higher reality within us and to cast aside all the superficial crap that we have allowed to clutter up our lives. In confronting a potentially fatal disease, we are led to confront our deepest selves. If we fail to do this, we are running away from our own source of strength, our Healer Within.

A lot of what I write in this book may seem fairly self-evident; other parts of it may lead you into new realms of experience and understanding. All that I ask is for you to suspend that rational, judgmental side of you and just accept what you *feel* is right.

This book is divided into four parts:

1. *Body, Mind and Spirit* focuses on the physiological systems which maintain balance within the body and shows how these are related to energy centres which are the seat of our emotional and spiritual selves. Particular emphasis is placed on the need to turn away from the means of transmission and the symptoms of the virus, and instead to focus on the deep, underlying cause of the state of imbalance which allows AIDS to take hold within the body.

2. *Letting Go* is the central core of the book. Illustrated by case studies of people with AIDS, it identifies the main causes of deep imbalance within people with AIDS and shows how these can be released and let go.

3. *The Healer Within* focuses on the true essence within all of us which, if expressed and fulfilled, will banish any disease from our bodies and much more.

4. *AIDS – A Broader Perspective* explores the ways in which AIDS is a disease reflecting the changes which humanity as a whole is going through on a spiritual plane, and how we can use the experience we have undergone with AIDS to transform our own lives, as well as helping others to transform theirs.

In case these chapter descriptions seem a little vague, do not worry. The whole point of this book is that it should be used as a workbook rather than just a book of theory. As you go through the various stages, there is a whole series of guided meditations to lead you into a deeper and more active understanding of how you can heal yourself.

Healing yourself: the essence of this message is responsibility. You are responsible for every aspect of your life and your health is just one part of it. If you take that responsibility into your own hands, then you can create health within your body. If you do not, then you are surrendering your power.

Please note. This book is not meant to replace medical treatment; it can be used in harmony with traditional medicine.

1

Body, Mind and Spirit

What is disease?

Health is balance and harmony; disharmony and imbalance lead to ill health and disease.

This may appear to be a very simplistic statement, but from it comes the essence of an understanding of the source of disease.

As long as we cling to the notion that our body is an isolated entity, just as the doctor often treats the symptoms of a disease rather than dealing with the root cause, then we shall never begin to understand what makes certain people sick and others healthy.

As I said in the introduction, we must go deep within ourselves. Forget about KS (Kaposi's sarcoma) or PCP (Pneumocystis carinii pneumonia) – they are simply the external symptoms of the disease we call AIDS, like the tip of an iceberg. Things have been going on a long time in your body before such outer signs manifest themselves.

O.k., so, you have a virus – say the AIDS virus, the HIV virus or whatever name you wish to call it.

In itself it is a living organism – it has evolved into a highly efficient organism, feeding on the very system within the human body which should destroy it.

Yet, it is important to understand that of all living organisms on this planet, man is the most highly evolved, whilst a virus is one of the simplest forms of life on earth. Why is it, therefore, that such a microscopic, simple organism is capable of destroying this amazingly complex and efficient structure that is the human body?

Or, to put it another way, why is it that some who are exposed to the virus get sick and others do not?

On a physical level, it is all to do with the immune system and its effectiveness. If the immune system is in 100 per cent working order, then the virus will be detected and destroyed; if it is out of balance or impaired, then the virus will be gradually allowed to establish a hold in the body until it is seemingly 'too late'.

Yet, the immune system itself is kept in balance by other systems within the body and it is these that form the mind/body connection that so many people talk about – systems so powerful that it is absurd to dwell on such words as 'too late' and 'incurable', as they are able to return the body to a state of perfect balance, just as they were able to undermine that balance in the first place.

This is the essence of the Healer Within and the aim of this preliminary chapter is to give you a basic understanding of the physical workings of this process.

The Endocrine System

Homeostasis is the medical term used for the intricate balance that is maintained within our physical bodies. From the simplest physical reactions to the most complex thoughts, it is the co-operation between the millions of microscopic cells within us that keeps us functioning throughout every second of our earthly existence – just as a beehive cannot survive without the unified purpose of all its members.

The two primary systems which are responsible for maintaining this homeostasis are our nervous and endocrine systems. It is on these which I now wish to focus.

Just close your eyes for a moment and concentrate on that very central part of yourself which runs from your brain down to the very base of your back – this is of course your spine and wrapped around it is your central nervous system.

There are three kinds of nerves, all of which are connected to the brain through the spinal cord: the sensory nerves which bring our sensory perceptions into the brain; the motor nerves which send signals from the brain to our limbs etc., and the autonomic nervous system which maintains regular nervous functions such as the beating of the heart. All three are essential to the maintenance of balance within the body by instantly sending messages between the brain and any part of the body which is threatened by imbalance.

The endocrine system works in tandem with the nervous system and, by the particular way it works, is the most essential system for maintaining balance or homeostasis in the body over the long term.

Unlike the nervous system which sends messages rapidly to its target organs, the endocrine system works by a much more slow moving process. It operates through chemical messengers or hormones which circulate in the blood and modify the activity of the various vital organs throughout our bodies. It is a change in the body's internal or external environment which initially triggers the release of these hormones into the bloodstream; once balance has been restored, a process called 'biofeedback' occurs, whereby this balance is conveyed back to the initial point of control and the secretion of the hormones ceases.

Hormones are stored in and released from the endocrine glands and it is on the ones relevant to this book which I shall now focus, not just in a purely physiological sense, but their effect on the broader aspects of balance within us.

The pineal and pituitary glands: The pituitary gland is known as the 'master gland', as its activity controls many of the other glands beneath it in the body. It is linked, through the hypothalamus, to the brain and thereby to the central nervous system.

Virtually nothing is yet known by modern science about the pineal gland, which is situated in the brain above the pituitary gland. In fact, the pineal gland is the 'inspiration' of the endocrine system, transmitting many messages to the rest of the body, sometimes through the pituitary gland, sometimes by-passing it.

The thyroid and parathyroid glands are located in the throat; they are responsible for metabolism and the regulation of our physical and mental growth.

The sex glands – the testes in men and ovaries in women. Aside from their obvious reproductive function, they also have considerable influence on those less physical aspects of us which we call our moods and emotions.

14

The Thymus and the Heart Centre

It is very sad how the thymus gland is so very much misunderstood and so totally underestimated. If there is one part of the first chapter that I wish you to firmly implant into your mind, it is this one, as I shall be referring again and again to this section of the body and, in particular, what it represents on a level that has implications far beyond the purely physical.

If you read any text book on physiology, this vital organ will be given barely a paragraph. It is known that this is where the T-cells mature within the unborn baby and also that it shrinks as a child reaches puberty. Because it becomes smaller at this age, it has long been presumed that it no longer has any real function in the human body after adolescence.

They could not be more mistaken. You only have to look at the size of the thymus in the body of a person who has died of AIDS to fully understand how shrunken the thymus can become when a person's immune system has been totally wrecked.

In a healthy adult, however small it may be compared with pre-adolescence, the thymus gland, in association with its neighbour the heart, is *the regulating system of the whole immune system*.

It will only be a matter of years before scientists fully discover the extent of this, and, indeed, discoveries are already being made to point in this direction. (An excellent book which establishes this in a scientific, empirical manner is coincidentally also entitled *The Healer Within*, published by E.P. Dutton, New York.)

The thymus lies at a point level with the heart, roughly where the heart would be if it were centrally located. It is at the focal point of the Heart Centre, about which you will be reading much more later on.

The heart is, as we all know, associated with love, and how many of us have heard the old saying: 'Love heals'?

The Adrenal Glands and Stress
I'm going to start this section off with a story.

Imagine that you are a stone-age man walking along by yourself and you suddenly come face to face with a sabre-tooth tiger. You freeze and in an instant make the decision whether to flee or stand and fight. The outcome is simple: either you escape or kill the tiger or you end up as a tasty meal.

This in a basic way illustrates what is called the 'Flight or Fight Syndrome', which is closely linked to our adrenal glands. When we are confronted with something like the sabre-tooth tiger or, in other words, when our brain receives the signal that there is some outer threat to ourselves, our adrenal glands, which lie perched on top of our kidneys, secrete certain hormones which direct most of our energy to the outer limits of our body, our limbs. This is done in association with messages sent from the brain to the motor nervous system. When the threat is past, then, through a system called biofeedback, normal balance is restored.

The 'Flight or Fight Syndrome' is also associated with that vague concept we call stress.

Stress, in a physiological sense, is exactly what it says. If you build a footbridge, the iron girders with which it is built are chosen because they are strong enough to carry the anticipated weight load of the bridge indefinitely. If, however, it was suddenly decided that this bridge would be used by cars and trucks, then the stress on these girders would be greater than what they were built for and one of them would finally give way, leading to the collapse of the whole structure.

Well, stress within the body is no different. The human body is built to live in a reasonably stable environment with emergency systems built in to react against periodic shocks from outside. In the case of the sabre-tooth tiger, or, for that matter, a 400-metre sprint, the body increases its output of energy. When it is over, the body slowly returns to normal.

So-called 'emotional stress', on the other hand, is a completely different matter. Most of us in the West are fortunate enough to be living in a society in which physical threats to our lives are rare. Yet, such is the way that 'civilized' man has developed that he has allowed other factors to impinge upon his life and upon the emotional stability of his being. Some of these, such as the death of a spouse or relative, are at some time in our lives inevitable, but there are of course many other causes of stress.

Whether stemming from work, relationships or whatever, the physiological result is the same. Any emotional reaction has an immediate effect on the body – a simple example is of an angry man who goes red in the face – yet, as in the case of the sabre-tooth tiger, a short-term emotional outburst does not necessarily do any harm to the body. After the fact, the body returns to normal.

How many of us, though, are the type who express emotion and, in doing so, immediately release it? Very few, I suspect, and it is this inability to let go of an emotional experience which causes most damage to our bodies.

Let us return to the girder again. If, for instance, just one car is allowed over the bridge, it may groan and bend, but, once the car has passed over, the bridge will be in no immediate danger of collapsing. If, on the other hand, cars will continue to cross the bridge *ad infinitum*, the weight of each car will have an accumulative effect on the girder until it can finally take no more and collapses.

The human body is of course an infinitely more complex organism than an iron girder, but the same process occurs with long-term stress within a human being. When there is an element of emotional stress within a person's life, the brain perceives it in the same way as it perceives any threat to the entity which it controls, and sends out messages to counter any effect it has upon the body. As with physical stress, it is the endocrine system, and the adrenal glands in particular, which do most of the work, secreting hormones to deal with any imbalance that may have occurred on a cellular level.

However, there is a fundamental difference between the working and effect of physical and emotional or mental stress. Whereas physical stress is almost always relatively short-term and can be identified through the nervous system as coming from a specific location, non-physical stress can be carried around unresolved for huge stretches of time and cannot be identified as coming from a specific physical location.

So, put in a very simple way, what happens when we carry unresolved stress around with us, our body is searching for something it cannot specifically react to and is therefore always on red alert, using energy for nothing. Or, more to the point, the natural balance within the body, homeostasis, is disturbed and all of the major functions which maintain health within the body are impaired. And of course the immune system is one of these.

Although I have used the word stress throughout this chapter, it is really too general a term. Just as I have explained its effect on the body in a very basic, simplified manner, I have used the word stress to cover a whole host of influences on our lives. Throughout our lives, there are things that happen to us which cause us suffering – some of us put the suffering behind us, accepting that this is a part of life, a means of learning and growing; others, indeed most of us at some point in our lives, hold on to the emotion behind the experience and allow this to fester within us, often quite subconsciously. Many of us will continuously carry around with us worries about work or a relationship, but there are far deeper rooted emotions and experiences which we carry around with us and of which, in our day to day lives, we are not consciously aware.

The bulk and most important part of this book focuses on the identification, understanding and, finally, release of these elements within us which I have described here as stress and which are the primary causes of imbalance taking root within our bodies.

Body/Mind

In the previous chapter, you will have noticed that, even as I talk about the physical nature of the body, I continually deal with non-physical matters. This is quite simply because the mind and body are inextricably interrelated. Anyone who tries to view disease in any other light only limits himself. This book is not about dealing with symptoms and trying another new drug to make the PCP or KS go away. It is about getting to the true source of sickness.

Nothing in the previous chapters, aside from what I wrote about the thymus, is in the least bit controversial. Even the most conservative doctor acknowledges that the state of the mind has an effect on the state of the body.

However, the remainder of the book is meant to lead you into realms and ideas that you may never have confronted before. A lot of what I have to write here will seem fairly obvious to you; certain things I write may not rationally appear to make a great deal of sense, but may just feel right; others may seem perfectly irrelevant to you. This book is not meant to be all things to all people; its purpose is to enable you the reader to recognize and to delve into certain parts of yourself that you have not dealt with before, and, in doing so, understand a little more about balance, harmony and health on the one hand and imbalance, disharmony and sickness on the other.

It is a fine dividing line and each of us has the capability to determine which side we remain on. If you are healthy, you can ensure that you remain so; if you are not, the transformation towards good health is within your own power.

Moreover, it is quite literally a question of choice. No true healer will ever say that it is he or she who heals a patient. As a healer, I act as a channel so that the people who come to see me may feel their own power within themselves. It is then up to the individual whether he or she draws upon that inner strength to get better. If you are resigned to death or you expect something or somebody to cure you, then death will come to you. If you really wish to live, to grow and to experience a new life, then there are no limits apart from those you impose upon yourself.

Everybody at some point in their life has gone through a period of emotional suffering, isolation or loss. We would all like to think that we don't have to go through any more such periods of hardship – yet, when you look back, these are also the periods when we learn most about ourselves and grow. It may sometimes even seem as if it is only by suffering and having to endure pain that we are taken off the day to day treadmill of our existence and are really brought face to face with our inner selves.

The reason I mention this is that you are presumably reading this book because you have undergone the pain of having been diagnosed with AIDS or you are frightened that you will be coming down with AIDS. In either case you are confronted with your own mortality and all the fears that this brings. AIDS represents the greatest challenge in your life.

Well, let me tell you one thing. Of all the many people I have met who have come down with AIDS, there is one common thread that runs through all those who have survived a long time and remain in a stable condition. They have all taken their lives into their own hands and have lived them to their fullest. Many have recognized that, before they became sick, there was a great deal wrong with their lives – not in a moral sense, but quite simply that their day to day existence gave little satisfaction and fulfilment, that there was a deep feeling of emptiness in their lives.

Many of these wonderful people have said to me that the quality of their lives has actually improved since they were diagnosed.

Is that not remarkable? That this disease which has cast so much pain and fear across the world can actually produce something positive in our lives?

But then, it is not so strange, because AIDS is much more than just a physical virus; it has become so enmeshed in our consciousness that it has assumed proportions beyond those of other diseases which afflict the world. And where there is emptiness within our own consciousness, our own inner selves, then the AIDS consciousness finds space to enter into our being.

I know that for many of you this concept may appear a little far-fetched, but the following chapters will enable you to see how easily we can allow ourselves to give up our power to entities which should have no power over us; and, on the other side of the coin, how easily we can reclaim that power within ourselves.

AIDS need not be the end. It can be and already has been for certain people the beginning of a new life where they understand that there is a potential within them far greater than they had ever realized. The Healer Within is just part of that potential.

What I am going to ask you to do is to start looking at your life in a new way, one in which you recognize that it is your right to lead a fulfilled existence based on peace and joy, warm and loving relationships and a freedom to create your own reality.

I'm going to ask you to cast aside that part of your upbringing that teaches you that you must prove yourself, accumulate possessions around you, compete against others, conform. And, in its place, all you have to do is follow your intuition, your conscience, what you *feel* is right.

Our True Essence

The reasons I have focused so strongly on the endocrine system are twofold, both interconnected. Firstly, there is the physiological function of maintaining balance within the body. Secondly, and of equal importance, these physical glands are directly linked with non-physical energy centres which are every bit as real as the endocrine system, although they cannot be seen on a physical plane.

Every human being has seven of these energy centres (in fact, many more, but I work only with these seven) and each one relates to a part of what may be called the psychological or spiritual side of us. We are not just flesh and blood; we have a consciousness. We question things, we can express and feel things – although all this is put down to the function of the brain on the physical level, we are all beings of spirit and aspirations far beyond our physical limitations. How otherwise can you account for the importance of love in our lives? Do you really believe that this is purely a function of the body?

As our so-called intelligence has increased, our society has come to rely on what can be proven, what can be understood by our rational mind. All else is often considered irrelevant. There was a time when religion fulfilled that part of man which reached out towards a higher reality, but organized religion has become so obsessed with dogma and sin that much of the true sense of spirit has gone out of it.

What do I mean by spirit?

All of us have at some time felt a yearning for something higher within ourselves and our fellow men. We have most of us at one time stood at the top of a mountain or on a deserted beach overlooking the wide expanse of ocean and felt something surge through us that cannot be explained in material terms.

That is our true essence, for the sense of awe and wonder we feel puts us in touch with the limitless energy of which we are all part. Whether we call it Nature, the Universe or God, it does not matter. It is there around us and it is also there within us to draw upon whenever we need it.

And if this seems somewhat unrelated to AIDS, then just see AIDS as a gigantic kick up the ass. If the questioning, pain and fear that AIDS has brought into our lives is not enough to make us truly confront the essence of ourselves and cast away all the shit that we have allowed to build up around us over the years, then I wonder what will.

Which brings me back to the seven energy centres or chakras, which is what they are called in the East. In the East, and even in the ancient civilizations of the West, these chakras have always been the focal point of healing activity, as it is through them that the activities of the mind and the inner life of man work through into his body.

When someone who is sick comes to see me, it is the blockages within these centres that I see or rather feel; or, to put it another way, I become aware of exactly what it is within the inner life of the person which has so drastically thrown the vital systems of the body out of balance. It is only through the recognition and understanding of the source of this imbalance, often hidden deep within the subconscious, that I can start to work with a patient in restoring his or her inner life to its original state of balance and harmony. As this harmony is created within the chakras on the etheric plane, it gradually filters through the endocrine system, creating balance in the vital organs of the body.

But, before I go on to explain the specific links between the chakras and the endocrine system, one word of warning. It takes years for us to accumulate all the experiences and attitudes which we allow to take power away from our inner selves, our essence, just as it takes years for the HIV virus to take hold within the human body and to develop into fully-fledged AIDS. If it takes so long for imbalance to occur, then balance cannot be restored in an instant. In order to activate the Healer Within, you must first acknowledge the potential within yourself; then it is a matter of discovering that potential as you go deeper within yourself, like peeling away the layers of an onion. Patience is not in great supply in our fast paced world but, for a venture of such great significance, it is a great ally.

The Seven Chakras

Before I explain what part of us each of the chakras represent, it will do no harm for you to visualize them.

As I asked you to do earlier in the book when talking about the central nervous system, just close your eyes for a few moments and focus on that central part of yourself which is your spinal cord running from your brain down to the base of your spine where you sit down. It is along your spine that the chakras are situated, the first pointing downwards, the seventh upwards and the five in between out in front of you.

In order to visualize them, see in your mind's eye the shape of a cone, or more specifically a swirling energy in the shape of a whirlpool or the eye of a tornado, with the narrowest point fixed in the spinal cord and the widest point coming about two inches out from the body. It does not matter if you have problems with visualizing this – this is just at this point to give you a physical point of reference, as I now focus in on each one individually.

The First Chakra is situated at that very point of the base of the spine called the coccyx bone, where you sit down. Pointing downwards from this point, it is your connection to the earth, your basic instinct for survival, your 'common sense'. It is also through here that there is a special connection between a child and its nurturing parent, usually the mother. It is not connected to any part of the endocrine system.

The Second Chakra is situated two fingers below the navel and points outwards in front of the body. It is the seat of EMOTIONS, SEXUALITY, CREATIVITY and, as it happens, psychic capabilities. It is connected to the sex glands within the endocrine system.

The Third Chakra is located in the solar plexus, just below the breastbone. It is the centre of POWER and STRENGTH, which may see very vague terms, yet you will see in the next section of the book how important this chakra is. It is connected to the adrenal glands.

The Fourth Chakra is on the level of the heart but, unlike the physical position of the heart, is along that central line down which the spinal cord runs. It is often called the Gateway to Heaven, as this marks the beginning of the 'higher' aspects of man. It is the centre of LOVE and COMPASSION and is connected to the thymus gland.

The Fifth Chakra is located in the throat and is the centre of COMMUNICATION and EXPRESSION. Because creativity and emotions have much to do with this centre, there is a strong link between this and the second chakra. In addition to this primary chakra, there are subsidiary chakras attached to it which are in the hands, particularly the palms and the fingertips. This chakra is linked to the thyroid and parathyroid glands.

The Sixth Chakra is the renowned Third Eye just above the eyebrows. Here is the seat of our INTUITION and CLAIR-VOYANCE, as well as the RATIONAL MIND. It is connected to the pituitary gland.

The Seventh Chakra is at the top of our head, our Crown, and faces upwards. It is our direct, personal link to the universal energy that I have talked about, or God, or whatever you wish to call it. It is our ultimate guiding force and brings all the other six chakras together as one. It is connected to the pineal gland.

You will note that the two chakras on each end of the spectrum point upwards and downwards, while the others point outwards in front of the body. This is because they relate specifically to the two fundamentals, the duality, of our essence: the physical and the spiritual.

Yet, although they seem to be on the opposite ends of the spectrum, they are actually not separate, but are part of the same substance which is that individuality within all of us. Just as our minds function much more effectively if we combine the rational and intuitive parts of our nature, so it is with these two apparent extremes, the physical and spiritual. If we can bring them to work in harmony with each other rather than flitting from one to another, as we all have a tendency to do, this is a great step towards achieving harmony in our lives.

It may interest you to know that all the most powerful spiritual beings, teachers and healers that I know of my generation in their thirties are also the most sexual beings I know!

Much of what I write in the main section of this book is to teach how these seemingly distinct parts of our nature can be brought into harmony with each other to create the balance we need to maintain health in our bodies and prosperity in every aspect of our lives.

But before progressing to this most vital part of the book, I wish to explain a little more about that physical part of us and how we can draw upon the energy of the very earth we stand on.

The Physical, the Earth and the First Chakra

When you lay sick in bed and you are racked with discomfort and pain, there is an overwhelming feeling of being 'trapped' within your body. This analogy is not very far from the truth, for, confined as we are within our physical form, we cannot escape the reality we create around us.

In this physical form, we are continuously bombarded by a whole host of outside forces throughout our lives – each thing we come face to face with we must confront or react to in one way or another. Sometimes, we try and shy away from some of the choices we have to make, but, in the end, the way in which we react to these major choices shapes the course of our life. There is no escape from this physical reality and the responsibility we have for our own lives. It is a law of the universe that all that we leave unresolved in our lives will at some point return to confront us again, albeit in another form.

This is why AIDS has proved to be such a powerful vehicle for change for so many people – it has forced us to stop racing around from one thing to another and confront the very essence of our existence.

Also, as physical beings in human form, we are an integral part of the planet on which we live. As our civilization has supposedly evolved and we have begun to see ourselves as separate from, even masters of, nature and the earth, so we have lost an understanding of the earth that many ancient cultures had – not just in terms of herbs and their benefic effect on the body, but how we can draw healing energy from the earth itself.

Just as all our cells are living entities unto themselves and are also an integral part of our body, so are we humans individuals unto ourselves and also an integral part of the planet earth; just as the earth is an individual planet unto itself and also an integral part of our solar system, and so on and so on.

What this means is that we are a fundamental part of a far greater whole, which has an energy that can be drawn on whenever we please, as long as we open ourselves up to feel it.

The way I explain this feeling is always to compare the inherent difference within me when I am in the country, rather than the city. Having been an urban dweller for the last half of my life, I have become very accustomed to the way my mind behaves when I am in the city. There is a continuous tendency for the mind to flit from one thing to another, as there are always so many possibilities, so many choices, so much going on. In the country, there is a greater sense of tranquillity, often too much so for the hardened city dweller!

But, the difference goes far beyond there being things to do and not to do. There is a fundamental difference in energy and the reason I am dwelling on this point has a lot to do with that dividing line between health and sickness. That difference is what is called *grounding*.

Let us return once more to that wonderful feeling which runs through you when standing on a beautiful deserted beach. There, standing upon the earth, you are taking in the whole scene with all your senses, not just the visual, and, in opening yourself up with that sense of wonder or appreciation, you are subconsciously connecting yourself to the earth. In reality, you are allowing that earth energy to enter into you through that first chakra, and the rush that you feel is indeed the healing energy of the earth.

If you are sceptical about this, just go to a favourite area that you associate with peace and tranquillity, whether it be in the country or a city park. Sit with your feet on the ground, just allow your mind to go blank and feel the energy of the trees and all around you just become part of you. I will lead you through a meditation to do this at the end of the chapter, but the most important thing is just being *aware*, opening yourself up to the pleasure of your senses all combined together.

AIDS is primarily an urban disease for the obvious reason that the two groups most at risk, gay men and drug abusers, tend to be concentrated in urban areas. But, there is another factor and that is the lack of grounding.

So many of the people I have worked with who have AIDS, in particular in New York, I see and feel very strongly as lacking that grounding element within them.

If you are constantly in an urban environment with concrete underfoot and all around, living fifteen floors up, one's contact with the earth is bound to be minimal. What this means is that there is little to counteract all the constant pressures and variety of an urban lifestyle, where the mind is always active and flitting from one thing to another: there is no base, no fundamental grounding point.

This leads once more to a state of imbalance. In a physical sense, it is as if you take a pyramid and try to make it stand on its apex instead of its base.

The reason I am taking pains to stress this point is that the people with AIDS whom I know who have that contact with the country, that feeling for the earth part of themselves have a much more tranquil inner strength with which to counter the disease.

That is why this is one of the first things I always touch on with people with AIDS. If you live in the city and you cannot get out into the country, then at least try and spend some small amount of time in a park each day and feel the earth beneath your feet. If this is something you almost never do, you may be very sceptical that it has any relevance whatsoever to your health but, if you try it with an open mind, you will ultimately come to feel the healing power that is within the earth.

This is a meditation which will enable you to focus your mind upon this energy. Although very simple, it is a very powerful meditation which I do every day – it is best done outside, but is equally well done at home. If you do it inside, sit comfortably but upright in a chair with your feet on the floor, close your eyes and just imagine, if you wish, that you are sitting leaning against a tree trunk, the sun beating down upon you.

MEDITATION NO.1

With your eyes closed, breathe deeply from your diaphragm both in and out, and, as you breathe, focus in on that central part of yourself which is your spinal cord – indeed, see your breath move up and down your spinal cord, slowly up and down.

Once you are comfortable with focusing on your spinal cord, you gradually see it extend downwards out of your body into the earth. You can visualize it in whatever way you want – you may see it purely as your spinal cord coming out of your body, as a bamboo, the root of a tree, a rope with a stone attached to weigh it down, anything as long as it is linking you to the earth.

Slowly, this extension of yourself, this grounding cord goes further and further down into the earth, and, as it does so, you can follow it down, through the various layers of the earth, the soil as we know it with all the living organisms inside, through the various layers of rock, liquid, gas, one on top of each other, deeper and deeper until you feel yourself reaching the hot, liquid core of the earth. And, as you descend, you feel its warm, nurturing quality envelop you.

Leaving this grounding cord rooted in the earth, you return to your body and focus on the soles of your feet, visualizing a small round opening appear in each of them. Then, from the depths of the core of the earth, you see two shafts of energy rising up towards you and entering into your body through these openings in your feet. And the earth energy that you feel is a warm, reddish-brown, heavy energy, almost like the lava that pours out of a volcano.

And this dense, nurturing energy fills your feet, works slowly up your calves, over your knees, expanding through your thighs, over your buttocks and genital area, coming to a rest at your pelvis, so that the whole lower part of your body is filled by this earth energy. Then, as this energy continues to flow, any excess pours back into the earth through your grounding cord from the base of your spine, so that there is a continuous cycle of energy from the earth, up through your feet and down back into the earth.

And then, still continuing to feel this connection to the earth, you turn your attention to the top of your head and see another opening appear at your crown chakra. As you do so, you see coming from some distant part of the universe, whether from the sun, the moon, a star or anywhere far beyond, a brilliant shaft of bright gold light, like a laser beam, shooting into the top of your head through this opening in the crown. And the quality of this energy is much lighter, less dense than the earth energy.

This bouncing gold light completely fills your brain sweeping away in front of it any worries, any dark spots that may have settled there. It fills up the whole of your head, over your eyes, ears, nose, mouth, flowing down over your neck and shoulders, blasting away any tension that may have built up there, and then down your arms to the tips of your fingers.

And the main shaft of this gold, vibrant universal energy shoots downwards into your heart and, as it does so, it blazes forth into the whole upper part of your body through your arteries, cleansing your blood, your lymph system, surrounding your T-cells with a protective ray of healing energy, cleansing your lungs, kidneys and liver, bringing light and balance to your nerves, and, as it flows through all your vital organs, all the dark spots within them, the viruses, whatever should not be there, are swept away with the light and down into the earth.

Then, just sit there a while, feeling those two different currents of energy flow through your body, so that every cell of your body is filled with one or the other: the dense, nurturing energy from the earth as far up as your pelvis and the bouncing, gold light from above, each radiating health and harmony throughout every part of you.

Finally, in your own time, slowly open your eyes and put your hands to the ground, letting any unwanted energies within you flow out through them.

This healing meditation is to make you aware of those two parts of you: the earthly/physical energy and the universal/spiritual energy. They are both equal parts of you and if you ignore one at the expense of the other, you upset a natural balance within you.

This is what I call the 'maintenance' meditation, not only because I do it very quickly every day, but also because it is necessary to ground yourself in this way before undertaking the other meditations within this book.

If you at first find it difficult, don't worry. Try again and use your own creativity. You may visualize things in a different way. As long as you follow the basic guidelines, just follow your own intuition.

One last word about meditating in general. If you find your mind wandering, don't fight it or be hard on yourself. If your mind wanders, be aware of the thought, just let it float away and gradually bring your mind back to focus on that central part of yourself, the spinal cord. If you get angry with yourself or impatient, then your mind will never settle.

The Nurturing Parent.
Before I finish this chapter on the first chakra, you will remember that I mentioned that this was the chakra through which we are attached as a child to our nurturing parent – not in a physical sense through the umbilical cord, but in an emotional, reliant sense.

A young child is dependent for its survival on its nurturing parent, usually the mother, and this strong link is a perfectly natural phenomenon. The cord from the first chakra is actually attached to the nurturing parent for the first four or five years of a child's life, but, as the child develops greater independence, this tie loosens and the grounding cord is established in the earth.

How this occurs and what it means is not for this book, but I am bringing this up in this chapter because of a phenomenon related to AIDS.

Most gay men have a particularly close tie to their mothers, but I have sensed and discovered in a couple of people with AIDS a very powerful mother/child relationship where the person's view of his mother had barely changed since early childhood i.e. a very passive relationship.

When I was working on the first chakra, this came through so strongly, because there was no link between the first chakra and the earth; a very indistinct energy was coming from another source. I discovered later that there was a great need within this person for love and approval from his mother, partly because of her ability to constantly manipulate him.

Parents will come up quite a lot as this book progresses, but what I want to make clear here is that, if an adult is still tied to his or her nurturing parent's 'apron strings', this means that he or she is not grounded. That connecting point with the earth is instead attached to the parent.

34

And I cannot stress this too strongly: if you are not grounded, you run the risk of any of your bodily systems going out of control, out of balance. You have, I am sure, known someone who has had some kind of nervous break-down or disorder. That is a typical example of an un-grounded person, someone whose mind whirs away without the strength of the physical side, the earth energy to coun-terbalance it. (c.f. the expression 'down to earth'.)

In many people, a lack of this grounding manifests itself in an external nervous condition, but, more often, it manifests itself less clearly by creating imbalance in the inner workings of the body, such as the immune system.

That is why I am very serious when I say: 'Be aware of the earth', especially if you intend to make changes in your life.

2

Letting Go

The Second Chakra

As mentioned previously, the second chakra is the centre of sexuality, emotions, creativity and, as it happens, psychic powers. (Being psychic is no big deal; we all are if we have the faith to recognize it!) Such is the importance of the first three with respect to AIDS that I will be putting a lot of emphasis on the way that each of them has the potential of throwing our bodies into a state of imbalance and thereby into sickness.

Likewise, when understood and realized to their full potential, they can be instrumental in restoring balance to your bodies.

In this section, we shall be concentrating on all the different elements of this second chakra with particular reference to experiences I have had with people with AIDS. It is always this chakra, combined with the third, which needs the most work, for, once we have cleared all the mess we have allowed to accumulate there over the years, it is a natural progression for us to follow the higher aspects of ourselves and really feel that limitless potential within us.

For, this is what this book is all about. It is about regaining ownership and responsibility for your own life, freeing yourself from all the influences and conformity of the past, being at one both with yourself and with the higher force to which you belong.

Sex and Sexuality

I want to make one thing perfectly clear at the beginning of this chapter: *sex has very little to do with AIDS.*

What? You say. It is a proven fact that AIDS is sexually transmitted.

Yes, I reply. It is true that semen and blood seem to be the primary vehicles for passing on the AIDS virus.

But, I repeat, AIDS is not necessarily caused by sex.

Let me explain.

Any physical infection must have a means of entering the body. Some, like the common cold, we breathe in through the air. Others we consume in the food we eat; others are transmitted through the bites of insects or abrasions in our skin. There is a whole host of means of transmission – sexual transmission appears to be one of the primary means for AIDS.

Yet, I repeat, AIDS is not necessarily caused by sex.

There are, literally, thousands of people who have received the HIV virus through sexual transmission, but have not and *will not* come down with AIDS.

Why? Again, we return to the question of balance. If the HIV virus, or any virus for that matter, enters into your body and your body is perfectly or even moderately well balanced, your immune system will be working at 100 per cent capacity and will quite simply destroy the virus before it has a chance to gain any grip on any cell within the body, in

40

this particular case the helper T-cell.

I repeat once more: if you have been exposed to the virus, this does not mean that you will get AIDS.

Likewise, if you get AIDS, it is within your potential to recreate balance within your body, to create more healthy T-cells, to arrest and finally reverse the progress of the virus.

If you are not by now prepared to believe this, I suggest you throw this book away.

I have at this point spent enough time writing about viruses, endocrine systems, etc. I am now leaving the physical body behind and am turning to the true source of the disease, of any disease: the emotions, the mind, the spirit. These three things are all just words we use to define things as best we can. They are all intangible, but they are what make up our consciousness, our very reason for being alive.

So, in this chapter, I am leaving sex as a purely physical act behind and shall now go on to the much more complex field of sexuality, firstly in general terms and finally concentrating on homosexuality and what it really means to be gay. AIDS has so often been labelled as a gay disease that it has struck at the heart of most gay men's lives. This stigma itself is enough to destroy a person's balance and must be redressed immediately. But, more of that later.

What is sexuality? So often, we confuse the physical act of sex with the notion of sexuality, and, in doing so, we do ourselves a great disservice.

You only have to look at the numerous nature programmes on TV to see that the sexual act in the insect and animal kingdom primarily serves as a biological function. It is for the most part a very short and peremptory act, quite distinct from all the associations we connect with sex in our own lives. We humans are not purely animal – we are creatures of consciousness and sexuality is a major part of this.

Sex in its highest form is the most wonderful expression of love and intimacy open to us. Do not forget this. We are physical beings and beings of spirit, and sex as an expression of love is the fusion of these two seemingly distinct aspects of ourselves. I do not need to tell you the incomparable feeling that overwhelms your whole being during those moments when it all comes together – moments which we will often try to recapture at a later date without really understanding deep down what made them so special.

The trouble is that, for many of us, especially men, the memory that remains is often of the physical aspect of sex, rather than the depth of feeling that lay behind it – especially so after the break-up of a relationship, when the feeling has so often turned to anger or sorrow, and all that remains is the physical memory.

Which brings me to that awfully judgmental word: promiscuity. How many of you have first started a period of so-called promiscuity in search of 'love', that feeling where you could lose yourself in the arms of another person? How many of you have had passionate affairs where the sex was so wonderful that all else seemed unimportant, until the novelty of passion wore off and you finally realized that you had little in common with your partner? And then, the merry-go-round begins again and you want to recapture the best bits that still remain in your memory.

There is nothing wrong in this, because sex is the most incredible opener in the world – how much more quickly you can get really deep into someone (no pun intended!) during a sexual encounter than otherwise. It can break down so many barriers instantly.

Yet, and this is where we come to the crux of the link between sex and AIDS, what matters is what sex really means to us, what it is exactly that we put into a sexual relationship or encounter.

Just think a little about the motivations and true emotions that lay behind sex for you. Then, be perfectly honest with yourself and mark below those which apply to you in one way or another. You can add others if you wish.

Sex is:

☐ An expression of love for one particular person.
☐ An expression of love, intimacy and warmth with any

person.
☐ A way of getting close to someone more quickly.
☐ A means of finding a lover.
☐ A way of overcoming loneliness, of filling a void, a need within yourself.
☐ An adventure: the thrill of a new encounter.
☐ A means of escape from the day to day reality of your life.
☐ A way of releasing pent up energy and tension.
☐ A way of proving your own self-worth, your own attractiveness.
☐ A means of exerting power or control over someone or having someone do the same over you.
☐ Getting your rocks off – a purely physical sensation.

Also, I ask you to be aware of what sex has meant to you in the past, what it means to you now and what you want it to mean to you. Do you now view sex as good or bad, healthy or unclean, a natural impulse or something that should be suppressed? All this is important for you to understand.

Now, I am going to give you a scenario of the life of someone just before he came down with AIDS and explain how this contributed towards the onset of the disease within him. I say that this is the scenario of one person's life, but I have seen this with many variations in so many cases.

Peter has had one major relationship in his life and a few minor ones, but, at this moment, he is alone. Deep down, he still yearns for the warmth, comfort and intimacy that relationships bring. He goes out to a bar – it does not matter if this is a gay bar or a straight single's bar – and he looks for someone to take home with him. And then, it seems that he is doing this rather a lot. He does not always meet somebody, and, even if he does, it does not necessarily satisfy him. In fact, the more he does it, the greater the feeling of emptiness inside him. Even so, he continues to go out, because the fear of loneliness is even stronger within him.

In short, it becomes a habit. After a while, he loses any expectation of lasting tenderness from any of these encounters. If he stays in at night, he has his collection of dirty movies, so that he can fantasize about his ideal, physical sexual experience. When he goes out, he goes looking for a certain type, and when he brings this type home, he sees his partner as a sexual outlet with whom he can play out his fantasies. Deep down, he regrets not being able to become more intimate, but he has got so used to projecting a certain image of himself that he is afraid of exposing any vulnerability.

And then, wham, he gets sick.

Of course, there is a lot going on within Peter in this scenario and most of it has the effect of causing imbalance in his life and within his body. Cumulatively, the effect is devastating.

Let me explain bit by bit.

1. First of all, there is that feeling of emptiness. We have all felt emptiness to a certain extent at some point in our lives and don't fool yourself: you can be doing something every moment of your waking life and still feel that emptiness. But, more of that in a later chapter. The emptiness that Peter is feeling principally derives from the fact that he is looking for someone to fill that void. In the end, it is sex, rather than a personal relationship that fills the void and then only for short spaces of time.

AIDS, cancer, any major disease feeds on that harrowing feeling of emptiness, of isolation. For those of you who have undergone periods where you have felt that there is nothing really within your life which is lasting and gives you joy, you know the havoc it wreaks on your moods and your body.

Where there is emptiness and indifference in your life, this means that you have lost a sense of your true essence, that consciousness that is your own. And where there is no consciousness, the AIDS 'consciousness' can enter.

2. Where sex becomes a habit for whatever reason and the sexual act is not a shared *feeling* with your partner, then you open yourself up to a whole host of energies. When you reach the point of orgasm and that incredible physical feeling engulfs the whole of your body and mind, your second chakra opens so wide that it engulfs the rest of your body.

The fusion between two people having sex is not purely physical: what actually occurs is that energies on a non-physical plane are exchanged between the two partners through the second chakra.

If the sexual act is part of something deeper, where you are giving and receiving warmth and affection to each other, that exchange of energies is also on a heart level and can only be positive.

However, in Peter's case, the warmth has gone out of the sex; he has lost a sense of the individual person with whom he is having sex and it is just as likely that his partner too will be seeing him in much the same way: as an image, as a means of fulfilling a physical desire.

What happens in such circumstances is that Peter is opening himself up to any negative energies that may be coming from his partner, just as he is giving any within himself to his partner. If this happens regularly, then the power of these outside forces builds up inside him, once more creating imbalance within him.

That is why I say: 'Be aware of what sex means to you'. Like attracts like and, if you are using sex for any other reason than a sense of intimacy and warmth, it is more than likely that your partner will be doing the same, feeding any imbalance which is already inside you.

3. Peter, in trying to attract a certain type, is essentially playing a game and putting a mask over his true self. But, this is no game, as the mask can take over and he loses touch with what is his true essence, the human loving part of himself. Then, fear sets in and he is basically afraid to show any vulnerability or express any emotion.

Then, those true feelings that we all have within us are trapped deep down and are left to smoulder, unacknowledged, unexpressed.

All of these traits of behaviour amount to a suppression of that true spirit of love and warmth that are not only fundamental to our being but also to our well-being. Think back to the link that I made between the thymus and the heart centre and you will understand that the suppression of that loving part of you means also the suppression of much more, including our immune system.

The way we relate to others is a reflection of the way we relate to ourselves and, in the long run, our bodies.

Through this example, I am trying to get over the most important message about the link between AIDS and sex:

AIDS is not here to teach us that sex, in particular gay sex, is bad. It is here to teach us to understand that sex is an expression of feeling, of our highest selves. If we choose to ignore that and abuse it, then it will rebound upon us.

If this at first seems a judgmental statement, just sit a while and ask yourself whether you ever really want to have sex which is not a true feeling of intimacy. Follow your own intuition.

And, while I am on the subject of judgment, where does that fit in? How many times have you heard that if people, gay men in particular, were not so promiscuous, AIDS would never be upon us. How much have you allowed the moral judgments of other people to affect you to the extent that you judge yourself?

I shall not dwell on this, as there is a separate chapter on guilt and judgment, but, once more, I say to you. Follow your intuition. If you have sex with someone, even a one night stand, and the communication and feeling were there, and it *felt* right, then there is no reason for judgment. If you feel guilt because of what the media, even your friends, say, you are surrendering your power to them. Quite simply, if you feel guilt after having sex for whatever the reason, forget it. Not only is it a waste of time, but it is also one of the most destructive emotions that exist; because of the way we cling to it, it is one of the prime culprits that creates imbalance within the body.

The essence of sex and sexuality is the expression of that warm, loving part of ourselves which is in itself our essence. The following short meditation is to make us feel the difference between the purely physical and the deeper aspects of our sexuality.

MEDITATION NO. 2

Just close your eyes, and, as before, focus on that central part of yourself. Then, focus on that particular area of your second chakra just below your navel and feel that whirlpool of energy that goes within your body. As you do so, see yourself come out of your body and shrink down in size so that you can walk in through that hollow space that is your second chakra.

When you walk into that space, you find yourself in a dark room. It is dark apart from a bright light in the centre of the room and, as you walk up to the light, you see an image of yourself there. And as you see yourself, you bring anyone else into the light and turn the scene into what is your ultimate physical, sexual fantasy. Forget about any emotional connection; let your purely physical imagination run riot and feel within you the sex getting hotter and hotter, the light getting brighter and brighter, so that you can see every detail as if in a mirror, until the energy becomes so intense that it explodes and, all of a sudden, it is over and the light is gone and darkness returns.

And, as you are in the middle of this dark room, alone, you see in a far corner a faint glow that had been overshadowed by the bright light. You gently walk over to it and, as you get closer, you see once more an image of yourself with someone, but, this time, it is a softer image and you are wrapped in the arms of your partner. The person whom you bring into this gentle glow is the one with whom you have had the most loving, warm and intimate sex and you see yourselves exploring and opening up to each other with tenderness and feeling, kissing, slowly making love, and, as you do so, this sense of warmth, of equally giving and receiving spreads to the area around your heart and you feel your heart centre opening up and expanding and expanding, sending rays of warmth and peace throughout the whole of your body until the physical image and the feeling of openness and intimacy become one within you.

Then, for as long as you want, you hold onto that image and sensation, letting it flow through the whole of your body, knowing that you can attract and create this for yourself, and, whenever you feel yourself being obsessed by the physical image of sex, you can return to this other warmer image, the true expression of yourself.

And, finally, you turn around and leave this room, return to your body and open your eyes.

Homosexuality and AIDS

Most of what I write in this book can apply to anybody, but, as AIDS has until now struck mostly gay men, there are matters I wish to address which are very specific to gay men.

In a strange kind of way, gay men start off with a very distinct advantage in life. When you realize that you are gay, this is something that you inately feel is right within yourself, yet it is more than likely that the society you were brought up in condemns the whole idea as being morally wrong and repulsive. For many gay people, coming to terms with this and finally accepting that being gay is a natural and integral part of you can be a very long and painful process. Yet, once this has been achieved, it has hopefully created within you an inate, questioning spirit.

What do I mean by this questioning spirit and how is it an advantage? When you know deep within yourself that something is right and you see society as a whole condemn it, then that knowledge, that feeling should make you question all judgments of society. And, if you always listen to that questioning spirit, that intuitive part of you that knows what is right *for you*, then this will give you the freedom to constantly make your own choices concerning your life.

Much has been written about gay oppression – it is no better or worse than the many other kinds of oppression that are the scourge of our modern society. But the most important thing to understand is that you are only oppressed if you allow yourself to be, if you surrender your power to an outside source. And, here, I wish to focus on the ways in which we do this, for, within gay men with AIDS, one of the most potent forces which have led to the destruction of balance within is a low self-esteem – often so deep under the surface that it is barely noticeable even to the individual himself.

We might as well start at the beginning, the first hurdle: one's parents. There are of course a 'lucky' few whose relationships with their parents have been so close and intuitive that being gay never presented a problem, but, for many gay people, the fear of rejection or rejection itself was an integral part of growing up and being gay.

There are so many variations on this theme. Some never to their dying day tell their parents and within that decision is the constant burden of living a lie and the fear that they will one day find out. Others make the choice to or are forced to tell the truth and the reaction may vary from outright rejection to seeming acceptance with negative remarks thrown in here and there.

Whatever the reaction, though, it is vital for every gay person to understand exactly how he or she now feels towards his or her family. Our parents are the symbols of nurturing love, even if you have had an unhappy childhood, and rejection, however slight, of any part of you as fundamental as being gay represents a withdrawal of that nurturing element. The result of it may be a smouldering anger, a sense of loss or, worst of all, an unacknowledged sense of being unworthy.

Even if you believe that you have resolved your relationship with your family, just put a few restful moments aside and really recognize and understand how you genuinely do feel towards them. If there is resentment, anger, pain or even guilt, just be aware of the emotion, I shall teach you how to release it later on.

Another negative factor that I have found cropping up again and again with people with AIDS has been religion, especially amongst Catholic and Jewish men. For me, this is particularly sad and pointless, as religion is supposed to be the focus of the spiritual side of man; but, so often today, religion is used as a tool and an excuse for hate and intolerance.

All I can say to those who carry deep within them an underlying guilt about being gay because of their religious upbringing is this: God is within you, each and every one of us is a divine being; but, most important of all, God is love. The essence of spirit is love and, if those immersed in the bigotry of what they call religion wish to impose their hatred on the world, you are only feeding this hatred if you take a feeling of guilt upon yourself. If someone says you are evil, that is their problem, not yours. It is their limited perception of you. It is not you.

And of course, the same applies to anyone who condemns homosexuality, from the popular press to the people you work with. It is they who have the limited vision and, if you accept this vision, however imperceptibly, you are limiting yourself. Understand that something you feel deep within your consciousness *cannot* be wrong. You are what you are.

Sexuality: the Male and Female Within Us

Jung was one of the first to fully recognize that every person, whether man or woman, gay or straight, has male and female within them – the terms he used were animus and anima respectively. He saw the ideal as being total balance and harmony between the two.

You will note that the words balance and harmony crop up again, which is why I am bringing up this particular subject in relation to AIDS. Everybody to a certain extent plays roles, often quite subconsciously because they appear to be the norm in our modern society. One of the most common of these 'accepted' roles is the way we assume the 'normal' behavioural standards of our sex, acting out our lives in a masculine or feminine way. Nowhere is this more evident than in 'macho' behaviour, which is in essence a fundamental denial of a whole part of oneself: the anima.

The animus within us is that part of us which is active, assertive and essentially rational; the anima is the passive, nurturing and essentially intuitive side of us. To say that one is the domain of man and the other the domain of woman is absurd, yet many of us have been brought up not to acknowledge the part of us which is not associated with our sex. This is of course changing, as women are allowed to have their own aspirations and goals and men are slowly permitting themselves to show the warm, emotional side of their nature. But, despite these changes, for many people, these old stereotypes still hold true.

The extreme animus character is the macho type who is dominant, aggressive, intolerant and unable or unwilling to express feeling; the extreme anima character is moody, indecisive, 'bitchy' and manipulative. Within both of them, the problem is exactly the same: the extreme animus completely denies and suppresses the anima part of him and *vice versa*. As with any suppression, the imbalance this causes sooner or later makes its way to the physical plane and affects the health of the body.

As I mentioned previously, there are certain inherent advantages to being gay and one of them is the greater ease with which gay people are able to recognize and appreciate the male and female within them. And yet, within gay society as a whole, how many people there are who, whether through fear of this duality within them or an acceptance of the need to mask their true selves, assume the outward behaviour of the two extremes: the 'macho man' and the 'bitchy queen'.

To those who choose to do so, I say: 'Understand what it is you are doing.'

Let us start with the macho image, which is quite simply projecting upon yourself the image of masculinity that you find attractive in other men, in the hope that they in turn will find you attractive. Such is the strong, predatory, sexual nature of the extreme animus that, where a man cruises another man, there is always a tendancy for this outer, purely sexual image to dominate. Once this develops into such a habit that it becomes ingrained within a man, the image becomes so dominant within him that he is afraid to let it slip, because, without it, he fears he will no longer be attractive.

What is particularly sad and ironic about this behaviour, which I have seen again and again, is that this mask is concealing a fervent desire to connect deeply with another man, a desire that can only be fulfilled by dropping the mask. And the longer this mask remains in place, the more a man loses contact with that feminine, loving side of him and the more the heart centre closes down, with all the ramifications this has regarding his health.

Fortunately, though, this is one of the easiest things to change, as long as you recognize it within yourself. Most of the people I know who have survived a long time with AIDS are those who have seen not only the absurdity but also the terrible strain of hiding behind a mask. They have made a conscious decision to no longer hide their emotions but to learn to share with other people their innermost feelings, to show the caring and nurturing part of themselves, their vulnerability, their desire for tenderness, affection and physical contact that is not purely sexual. And does this make them any less masculine? No way.

Leaving the macho image behind for now, I wish to touch briefly on the 'bitchy queen' personality and show how this denial of the animus, this extreme anima behaviour can have equal consequences for one's health.

The essence of this behaviour is the basic negativity that lies behind it. There can of course be great humour behind it, yet, even where this is so, the underlying current is one of putting out a negative, critical energy. There is also a great self-denigrating quality about this humour, which in moderation is fine, but, in extreme cases, can be very damaging. Just as the macho image can become ingrained into a person's being, so this seemingly superficial tendancy towards putting oneself and others down can root itself deeply within an individual.

What this extreme anima behaviour means is an underlying passivity which sees the fault for everything as being within other people and, most important of all, which sees everything as being beyond the individual's control. The end result is a situation whereby a person loses any sense of responsibility for his or her life, complains when things go wrong, but does nothing to deal with the source of any problem. With regard to AIDS, there can be a sense of resignation about it, as if it is 'something that was bound to come along anyway and there's nothing we can do about it.'

By focusing on these two extremes of animus and anima

behaviour, I am basically showing how much we lose by denying these two fundamental parts of our essence. Just for a moment think of yourself as a totally balanced being in this respect and feel the completeness within you. Think first of all of that receptive, loving part of you which values the warmth of human contact, the caring shown by real friends; then consider that active part of you, your own creativity and your ability to go out and create your own reality, express yourself in your own individual way. Then, just close your eyes and see yourself in harmony with the outside world, giving and receiving *equally*. There is no reason to deny any part of ourselves, and even less reason not to show to the world the way we truly are.

Emotions

I have written about some of the emotions that come into play with sex and sexuality, yet, of course, emotions are aroused by many different sources. What I intend to show in this chapter is how our emotions tend to relate back to very distinct individuals and events in our lives and how they can act as a dead weight around us, if we don't let them go. We can carry anger, guilt, jealousy, sorrow, fear and a whole host of other emotions around with us for a lifetime, but, if we do so, like an uncleaned wound, they can fester inside us and infect the whole of our body.

As mentioned earlier, all of us at some point in our lives have some period of intense suffering and pain or go through an experience which makes an immense impact upon us. These are generally the times of our lives when we become introspected and therefore learn most about ourselves. They also often give us the extra strength to deal with any other hardship that may come along.

Our emotions are nearly always wrapped up with the memory of such events and more specifically with particular people who have had influence over us. One of the consequences of our rational mind is that we have a tendancy to dart from the past to the future and back to the past rather than remaining in the stillness of the present moment. Retaining a memory of a bad experience is not totally a bad thing, as we have probably learnt from the experience. What does us harm, however, is holding on to the *emotional charge* of the experience.

I am often asked what I mean about emotional charge, so let me explain. Let us assume that I had been in a supposedly monogamous relationship for three years and my lover tells me that he or she has fallen in love with someone else and has indeed been having sex with that person for three months. Now, I had realized that our relationship had been coming to an end for a while, but it had just seemed too harsh a change to suddenly break it off and be alone again. So, when my lover tells me this, a whole host of emotions overwhelm me: anger at the dishonesty and betrayal; jealousy and hurt ego that my lover had gone off with someone else; sorrow and pain and a certain amount of fear and self-pity that I was now left alone.

Of course, deep down, we all know that 'time heals' and we ultimately recognize that a certain relationship was a transition period and was not meant to last, but many of us allow the emotional charge of the experience of loss to obliterate this knowledge. Instead of understanding that such an experience was part of learning and growing, we sometimes hold on to the emotions which were left in its wake, and, as they lie simmering in the recesses of our mind, they become embittered.

We may often think that we have let go of this 'emotional charge', but then we behave in a certain way which demonstrates that we have not. Sometimes, this may manifest itself in a reluctance to commit to a relationship through the fear of being hurt again, or, on the other end of the spectrum, we may enter into a period of promiscuity in search of the warmth of human touch which we have lost. We may find ourselves being angered by certain behaviour in others, because it reminds us of someone who has caused us pain. The list goes on forever.

This is what I mean by holding on to the emotional charge of an experience. Just one major event or relationship in the past which has caused great pain or suffering can, if not released, start off a pattern within us which robs us of our own inner strength. By holding on to such an event, or more often the person associated with it, we are quite simply giving it power over us. In particular, if the feelings involved remain unacknowledged and unexpressed, the pressure within grows and grows like the pressure that builds up gradually between two geological plates before an earthquake. And that earthquake could be anything in your life. It could be AIDS.

To illustrate this, let me give an example of a person with AIDS who came to see me once. The first thing I immediately became aware of within him was an immense anger that had obviously built up over many years. I told him what I felt and he vehemently denied that he felt any anger towards anyone in his life.

So, I went on to other things that were relevant to him and gradually edged my comments around to his parents. Suddenly, the floodgates of resentment opened. Out poured a whole history of conflict and some particularly devious and persistent behaviour by his parents that was designed to keep him under their power.

'So, you don't feel any anger then?' I asked him. 'I've never really thought of me being angry. I resent them, I suppose', came the reply.

It's funny how we can play games with ourselves, even with words, but all it means is that we so often bury things deep within us. There is of course nothing new in this, as any psychologist will tell you, but the way in which we consciously or subconsciously deny fundamental parts of our being and, in doing so, give them power over us, not only affects our behaviour but also the strength within us that enables us to maintain health within our bodies: the Healer Within.

In this particular case, the unresolved resentment towards his parents filtered through into every aspect of his life: nothing or nobody was ever quite right. If something bad happened to him, it was just bad luck, it wasn't fair; it certainly was not anything of his own doing. And, deep down, he felt that if anyone was going to get AIDS, it was bound to be him.

Quite simply, he had surrendered his power to the extent that, even when he recognized this, he went from one treatment and nutritionist to another, doing everything but look for the strength within himself.

Now, this may seem to be a very harsh and judgmental portrait of a person with AIDS, but if we all look deep within ourselves, most of us will recognize how, to some degree, we have or still do allow a certain experience or person in our lives to remain as a blockage within our inner selves. Anger is often the easiest emotion to recognize because of its explosive energy and is therefore the easiest to deal with, but there are many other less obvious and often more insidious ways in which we react to so-called negative experiences and influences in our lives.

I shall deal with these in a moment, but what is this rather vague notion of releasing that I keep mentioning throughout this chapter? It's all very well to recognize within you what is throwing your system out of balance, but how do you let that go and allow that harmony within to be restored?

Forgiveness

Quite simply, forgiveness is the most powerful weapon you have in your inner armoury, as it is forgiveness which breaks the hold which any negative emotional attachment from the past has upon you. Yet, for many people, forgiving is the most difficult thing to do, and I am talking just as much about forgiving oneself as forgiving others.

There are many reasons for this. Sometimes, it is pride or, an extension of this, the 'martyr complex', whereby we must show everybody how much we have been hurt. Indeed, there is a very strange contradiction within many of us that makes us hold on to a negative emotional state because it has become so much part of us that it is almost a comfort, a part of our personality that gives us security because it is familiar.

But, what really is forgiveness and what does it have to do with our health?

In simplest terms, and in its most important function as a restorer of balance, it is the release of any negative charge stored in the past; indeed, it is the release of any hold the past has upon us.

I have had many discussions with people, especially students and graduates of psychology, about the relevance of the past. For many psychologists, the past, in particular any negative patterns associated with it, is something first of all to be identified, then submitted to rational scrutiny, understood and to be 'made friends with'.

For me, the past is an encumbrance, excess baggage to be let go of. We are, each and every one of us, an accumulation of the experiences of the past – each major event in our lives makes its mark upon us and shapes us into the beings we are in the present, yet the past remains the past.

People who remain fixated in the past, whether on a negative experience or through a vague nostalgia for 'better times', must necessarily take energy and vitality away from the present life, and, when we are talking about sickness, we are talking about the present moment.

This is where forgiveness comes in. The more ingrained a feeling of anger towards someone may be within you, the more a sign of your own strength it is to forgive that person and let go of the emotional charge associated with him or her. By not forgiving and by holding on to the resentment, you are giving that person power over you, the last thing you really want to do.

Now, of course, if you have made a habit over the years of harbouring emotions deep within you without expressing, releasing or even recognizing them, it may well seem easier said than done to let go of them just like that. I shall be going much deeper into this problem in the later chapters on power and control, but, for now, I am offering a very simple meditation through which you can visualize and effect the breaking of the bonds between you and another person.

Remember. It is the cycle of life: as you forgive, so will you be forgiven.

MEDITATION NO. 3

Once more, close your eyes and focus in on that central part of yourself and breathe gently until you are at peace within yourself.

Then, focus on that area of your second chakra, just two fingers below your navel and imagine a cord attached to you at that point and this cord stretches off into the distance.

You then see yourself take hold of this cord and pull it in, and, as you do so, you see, attached to the other end, a person who has hurt you in the past and towards whom you still feel some attachment, whether one of regret, resentment or whatever. It can be a member of your family, an ex-lover, the one individual you associate strongest with inner pain and resentment.

As you see this person standing in front of you, you ask him or her: 'Why is it that you are still attached to me? What is the contract between us?'

You then wait for the answer to come to you. It may come from the image of this person in front of you or it may come from your own inner voice, telling you what the experience between you two taught you or what it was within this person which made he or she behave in this way or what it was in your own behaviour that brought out a negative response in the other person. Just take your time in this place of quietness and allow this person and the attachment between you to become clear, unencumbered by any emotional response within you.

Then, see yourself taking this figure in front of you by the hands and saying out loud: 'You no longer have any hold or power over me. I forgive you for all that you have done to me in the past, as this is no longer part of me, and I ask you to forgive me for anything I may have done to hurt you. I release you to your highest good, just as I ask you to release me to mine.'

Then, you quite simply tug at the cord that is attached to your second chakra and it comes away easily in your hand. You let go of it and it drifts away, together with the person at the end of it, into the distance out of sight. And you fill the gap left by the pulled out cord with a ray of bright gold light in the knowledge that this cord can never attach itself there again, drawing vital energy away from you.

Now, it is of course possible that you cannot find someone at the end of this cord and, if not, I suggest that you search deeply, as we all have some resentment towards someone and the least recognized can often be the most powerful. If you still cannot find anyone, good for you. If you do and you find that you cannot let go, just feel how much power you are allowing this person to have over you. Then, try again!

Guilt

I mentioned just now how much more difficult it can be to forgive oneself than to forgive others, and this leads on to this most destructive and most pointless of emotions: guilt.

'Don't be so hard on yourself!' How often have you heard that said? In this modern world, where we are brought up to achieve, to reach the highest standards (whatever they are supposed to be), how common it is to see people driving themselves crazy to meet a set of goals that have little to do with their inner selves, but are merely imposed upon them by pressure from parents, peer groups or society in general. The pressure to conform is enormous and failure to live up to certain so-called 'standards' results in one or both of the two main forms of guilt: self-judgment or assumption of other people's judgment.

In many ways, these two are one and the same thing. When I say assumption of other people's judgment, what I mean is the way in which we are constantly bombarded by the judgment of others over some aspect of our behaviour to such a degree that we come to assume a feeling of guilt over it. Self-judgment of course comes from the same source, but, for many, self-judgment itself is an addictive pattern, born from a need, instilled from an early age, to constantly prove oneself, to perform above the standards of others.

Returning to the assumption of other people's judgment, the most common and deeply damaging instances of this with regard to AIDS are concerning homosexuality, promiscuity and drug abuse.

I have already written a little about guilt in association with being gay: the pressures to feel guilt are enormous from parents and family, from religion, from the press – the list goes on forever. Society – or, at least, society in the so-called civilized world – puts so much emphasis on what it considers to be deviance from 'normal' sexuality that anyone who is gay can hardly avoid putting an inordinate emphasis on that aspect of him which is his sexuality.

I have seen again and again people with AIDS who hide a deep imbalance within them because of guilt about being gay – and, most often, this is the case with those who outwardly appear to be most at home with their sexuality, because they are the ones who, whether consciously or subconsciously, bury this feeling of guilt deepest down within themselves, sometimes through fear of it being recognized, maybe through fear of confronting the source of this guilt.

An example of this was an Italian-American gay man who appeared to have everything going for him. He was very attractive and successful and he seemed to have a close relationship with his family, all of whom were practising Catholics. His family knew he was gay and had never openly disapproved. Their way of dealing with it was to ignore it – his mother would still continuously drop hints about him getting married and a barrier had developed between them to the extent that this 'close relationship' was constantly fraught with the inner tension of never expressing their true feelings. The 'silent' guilt, together with the guilt left over from a strict Catholic upbringing, literally tore this man apart, even as he portrayed the confidant, attractive exterior to the world.

Guilt is so powerful an emotion that it becomes a revolving circle from which it becomes more and more difficult to escape. In this case, the pressure would build up inside him so strongly that the only release would be for him to go on a sexual binge, and then the remorse would set in.

I am certainly not saying that such emotional pressure is

inherent in every gay man, but it does no harm to really consider honestly and deeply how you view your own sexuality, in particular in relation to other people's opinions and judgment.

And then, understand this. The fact that you are sexually and, even more important, emotionally drawn to someone of the same sex *cannot* be wrong, as nothing that you *feel* deeply within yourself can be wrong. Take time out to take stock of yourself and recognize that you are essentially a warm and loving being. It is the quality of your feelings that matters. What you feel deep within you is your true essence and to in any way judge that essence is the best way to get sick.

Your essence is your strength; this strength and the balance it maintains within your body depends on your living according to your genuine feelings, your intuition, rather than submitting to the judgment of people who do not care to know what is truly going on within you. By turning on or in any way judging that emotional, individual part of you that is your own true self, you are turning away from your own source of inner strength.

That is why guilt can kill.

When it comes to promiscuity, drug abuse or any other 'addictive pattern', the judgment of society is compounded even more fiercely by the judgment of self.

We all know that promiscuity or drug abuse do not arise just of themselves – there are conditions within our lives and experiences which lead us into repeating the same behaviour over and over again, of looking for a way to escape, however temporarily, from the reality around us, from the emptiness of our inner lives. Guilt is the best way to perpetuate such a condition.

How many of us have come down from a fix or left a one night stand with a feeling of emptiness, and even more important, with a feeling of remorse. 'Why did I do it? What did I get out of it but an instant thrill? Why am I so weak?'

The key question of emptiness will be dealt with in a couple of pages, and, without dealing with this, no addictive pattern can truly be put to rest. But, the question of guilt and remorse is almost as important in confronting the problems of addiction, because the harder we are on ourselves for these 'lapses', the more our self-esteem will slip and the more addictive the pattern will become. This is the way guilt works, for it puts energy into the object of its fury and, in doing so, gives it power over us, binding us even closer to our addictive behaviour.

I can at this moment hear that traditionally moralistic, judgmental side of you saying: 'One should feel bad about it. We know that no good can come from it.'

If you assume such a position, you have not learnt the lesson of forgiving yourself and letting go. If you want to break a habit of any kind, you must accept what was done in the past as being firmly locked in the past without blame, without being harsh upon yourself. If you wish to change, you will in time by understanding the root of your behaviour, letting go of the judgment and allowing your self-esteem to return. If you continue to play the role of the 'Lady of Perpetual Guilt', you will quite simply remain stuck in the condition you are trying to escape.

Guilt is such a pointless waste of energy.

MEDITATION NO. 4

As before, close your eyes and focus on that central part of yourself and then move down to the area of your second chakra.

This time, you imagine yourself coming out of your body, shrinking down in size and facing your second chakra as if it is a long corridor stretching out in front of you. You enter this corridor and walk down until you come to a door, over which is marked the word: GUILT. You walk into a room and stand in the centre.

What you are now going to do is bring into the room all those people who have imposed a feeling of guilt upon you, starting with your parents. See them standing in front of you and see how they have harboured expectations for you, and when you have 'disappointed' these expectations, notice how they have judged you and how you have assumed this mantle of judgment upon yourself. If this has never been the case with your parents, let this pass, but be aware of any instance that they have judged you.

Then, as they stand there in front of you, walk up to them, take them by the hand and say to them:

'I thank you for your opinion and your perception of me. What I do in my life is my responsibility and there are no "oughts" in this world. If I do something, it is I who takes the consequences and I do not live my life through the eyes of others. Therefore, I release any judgment that you have imposed upon me and I act according to my own conscience. I feel no guilt for not living up to your expectations.'

From this point, you can bring before you any other people, even symbols such as a priest or the press, and repeat the same process, letting go of the hold which each of them has over you.

Then, bring in front of you any people towards whom you feel guilty because of any hurt you may have caused them. Ask their forgiveness and feel the release of accepting this from them, as they take your hands and let go of the emotional charge between you.

Finally, bring a mirror image of yourself in front of you and ask the question: 'What aspect of your life, your behaviour, your character do you like least about yourself? Why is it that you judge this part of yourself?'

And, as you see yourself in these roles, you say to yourself: 'I forgive myself for behaving in this way and I no longer judge myself. If I repeat this behaviour, I shall not be harsh upon myself, but shall be aware of my actions, understand and let them go, until I no longer need to repeat these patterns of behaviour.'

If you are gay, say to yourself: 'Being gay is just one part of my essence, an integral part. The sexual and emotional attraction I feel towards people of my own sex is a healthy expression of that warm, loving and intimate part of me, which is my true essence.'

Finally, say to yourself: 'I do not deserve to be sick. Whatever may have caused imbalance within my body in the past I now release from me and I see myself as being worthy of a healthy and fulfilling life.'

As you stand in this room, you see all those people you summoned into the room, including the image of yourself, file out through the door, until you are left alone.

As you breath in the space of this room, you assert to yourself: 'I shall never again allow the feeling of guilt to enter my being. I shall act according to my own conscience and not allow the views of others to dictate my behaviour. I trust myself and know that I shall grow from any mistakes I make.'

With this assertion of your own inner strength and guidance, walk out of the room, along the corridor and gradually return to your own body and space.

Isolation

A couple of pages back, I touched on the emptiness that all of us have at some point in our lives felt, an emptiness that cannot be filled by a good job, a nice house, 'sex, drugs, rock 'n' roll', outer possessions or fleeting pleasure.

With all this so-called progress in the material world, what of our inner lives and, most important of all, our relationships with our fellow men?

The majority of AIDS cases in the Western world are for obvious reasons to be found in major urban centres. For the many people who have flocked to the big cities of America and Europe, there is no returning to the more closely knit small towns or suburban communities where they were brought up. The lack of privacy and freedom would for most habitual urban dwellers be too stifling.

Yet, the comparative anonymity of a major city can have a fierce cutting edge. How true it is that a big city can be the loneliest place in the world. How many times I have seen people with AIDS surrounded by millions of people but no real friends to turn to.

Even this is a matter of choice. It is one that many have not even confronted as being a choice and, in not doing so, they open themselves up to isolation and the emptiness that goes with it.

What do I mean by this choice?

Let me give an example of a gay man living in New York.

He was attractive and always popular. Whenever he went out to bars or parties, he was always in the centre of a crowd, never at a loss for someone to chat to. Then, suddenly, he came down with the pneumocystis, closely followed by KS. When this spread to his face, he stayed at home. To begin with, he received an occasional visit from friends, but, after a while, these dried to a trickle. Soon after, he had another attack of pneumonia and died.

One's first reaction to this story may be: 'How awful that all his friends deserted him when he was sick.' This would be to lose the point of what really happened, for it was an unconscious choice that he had made which led to his sickness in the first place.

How often I have seen people with AIDS who, living in a big city, have lots of acquaintances, but, when it comes to the crunch, have no real close friends. To allow oneself to be in this position genuinely is a choice of an individual – more often than not, it is an unconscious choice, a way of life which is so easy to slip into, especially when times are on the surface good.

And, of course, this is not only confined to the gay world.

Let us once more picture this man I have just mentioned. He would come back from work in the early evening and, after eating, he would often go out to a place where he would see familiar faces, be in familiar surroundings. But, what of the times in between, what of the times he was down or lonely and wanted a friend to sit down and talk to, or even the times he was in an up mood and wanted someone, not necessarily even a lover, to share those deepest inner thoughts, the changes he was going through? He would go out more and more so as not to confront his inner loneliness. He would chat with people, yet would always miss the true intimacy and sharing of a deep friendship.

People who have always had real friends upon whom they could always rely and *vice versa* may think this scenario a little unreal, yet it is not uncommon. What is so sad is that it is so unnecessary. One only needs a handful of close, intimate friends and, as long as you have an open heart, they are

71

naturally drawn towards you.

So, why do people choose to isolate themselves in this way, an isolation which can slowly eat away at the very heart of someone, leaving an emptiness that can barely be comprehended? And how ironic it is that those who feel the deepest sense of isolation are often those who to the outside world appear the least so, as they have perfected the mask of self-assurance so well.

To those who do feel a sense of isolation deep within themselves, I say quite simply: 'The game is up!' It is purely a matter of choice.

I know that there are certain rare individuals who choose a life or at least a period of isolation to focus in on their inner selves, but they are few. For the majority, take away the rest of the living population on this planet and life loses its purpose. We are here to relate to each other, to learn from each other, to have fun with each other. It is people who offer the variety and energy of life – we only get out of human relationships what we put into them.

But then there is fear. Shyness is a form of fear – maybe general lack of confidence, fear of rejection, even of intimacy, of really opening up your true self. Especially so in this instant world of singles bars where an opening conversation is loaded with innuendo, acceptance or rejection may come in the first minute, where you feel a need to project a certain image which has nothing to do with who you really are.

In this case, I'm not going to suggest a particular meditation. I'm just going to say: 'Get over it!'

Do you really want to play games with people or do you really wish to relate to people? I have so often heard people say that they feel out of tune with the world, but, if you project an image of yourself which is not truly you, how do you expect to attract towards you people who are of your energy?

It is all a question of openness and understanding that you deserve the highest and most fulfilling relationships. If you remain closed and convinced that you are not worthy, of course people will pick this up and stay away from you. If you are open and trust in your intuitive reaction towards people, the people of your energy will be drawn towards you. It is one of the very simple laws of the universe. Like attracts like.

Do you want to share your experiences and feelings with others whom you trust, so that they can also do the same with you, giving and receiving equally in harmony with each other and yourself?

Or do you choose to isolate yourself and allow to creep into you the emptiness which allows disease to take hold within your body?

Choose carefully.

If this seems harsh, remember that AIDS has no compassion.

But AIDS is here to teach us many things. I have met many people with AIDS who have found common ground with other PWAs, their sickness, their fear bringing them together.

Yet, even this is only the ice-breaker. There is so much further to go. There are so many layers to peel away, so many defences and preconceptions to let slip before two people can meet each other face to face, inner core to inner core, in trust.

And this is the most essential part of our lives: peeling away the layers of the onion and revealing our inner core, being true not only to ourselves but also to others. This is the meaning of love and intimacy, and love is the highest healing element available to man.

That is why I shall devote a whole chapter to our understanding of love in its highest and most powerful sense.

Sorrow and Grief

Closely related to isolation is an energy I have come across in quite a few people with AIDS who carry around with them a deep sense of sadness, sorrow and pain, which lies like a darkness in the recesses of their soul.

This is the very antithesis of anger with its bubbling fury and resentment. Anger is associated with the colour red, the fire boiling within, while the colour of deeply felt sorrow, which has often been carried around like a dead weight for many years, is black, lifeless, almost completely drained of energy, yet no less powerful a disruptive force within the body than the fieriness of anger.

Sadly too, there lies within these heavy souls a strange sense of resignation about AIDS or disease in general, such that I have heard the following statement: 'I always felt that, if anyone was going to get sick in my circle, it would be me.'

Such is the power of thought and of the depth of suffering that some people hold on to.

Most often, such inner pain is associated with a loss which has overshadowed every other event in a person's life. This can either be the early death of a parent or someone very close or the withdrawal of love by someone upon whom the person depended. In the latter case, this may be the end of a relationship, which in another person may have aroused anger and resentment, but, in this case, the person carries the deep felt pain stoically within.

The energy associated with this is the most extreme example of how holding on to the past can drain and suffocate the healing power within, for the will to live, the sense of joy in life has been eaten away by the feeling, often deep down and unexpressed, that it is their destiny to suffer, to experience sorrow and pain. It is a complete denial of any power within the self, a final surrender to the notion that the individual is at the mercy of cruel destiny.

In someone who has AIDS already, it is a pattern that needs to be immediately arrested, for the natural progression is for that hidden resignation towards sickness to be closely followed by a resignation towards death.

This 'darkness of the soul' hits me right between the eyes as soon as I encounter it in someone, but it is not always obvious to everybody because of the stoicism that often hides it. Indeed, the extent of it is rarely even understood by the person involved.

Often, it is betrayed by continuous self-deprecating re-marks, as in the case of a man with AIDS whom I saw on occasions. At this time, he had begun to form an attachment to a person who was outgoing and was doing a lot of work with PWAs. It was obvious that they were both very fond of each other, but each time I saw him, he would tell me that it was not likely to go anywhere because how could such an outgoing free-spirited person want to end up with someone who was such a mess as he was. Each time we met, he seemed to have put another obstacle in the path of the relationship developing.

It was apparent to me at an early stage that, quite a few years back, this man had had a relationship in which he had freely invested much of himself, only to find his partner walk out on him for another man. This was the most important relationship he had ever had and he immediately took it upon himself that his partner had left him because he was not good enough, and from that day on he carried around this im-mense burden that he would never be worthy of the best.

How easy it seems to be for man to carry the burden of the bad times along in his soul and to leave the periods of happiness and joy by the wayside.

I shall not dwell on any more examples of our tendancy to cling onto sorrow and pain, but shall move on to a particularly powerful meditation in which you can feel within yourself the difference between sorrow and joy, leaving you in no doubt which is your divine right.

MEDITATION NO. 5

As with the meditation on guilt, you centre yourself and then leave your body and face your second chakra.

You walk along the corridor until you come to a door and over this door is written the word: SORROW.

You open the door and enter into the room. As you walk towards the centre of the room, you see a young child there by himself, crying and you realize that this young child is yourself.

As you see this image of you as a child in front of you, you recall the first time in your life that you remember feeling deep sorrow and pain. It may be the separation from someone who was close to you or it may be that someone you loved deserted you when you needed them. Whoever or whatever it may be, bring this person in front of you and ask them why they had to leave you then. Even if you do not receive an answer, take them by the hands or hug them if you like, releasing the sorrow and pain with the words: 'I forgive you for leaving me and understand that the sorrow I felt is now in the past and no longer has any hold on me. I bless you and release you, just as I ask you to do the same for me.'

Once you have done this for the first time, see this image of you as a child gradually grow up and as it passes through the various stages of your life, through adolescence, the first 'broken heart', all the painful memories of the past, confront them and let go of the emotional charge that surrounds them. Do not also forget to bring into this room and release those who have told you that sorrow must for whatever reason be part of your life and if one of those people is yourself, then release this image of yourself too.

Continue this until finally the figure opposite you is you as you are now.

There is no need to hurry this. Do not leave any stone unturned. Be aware of the strength of emotion surrounding each sorrowful experience and allow this to dissolve into thin air, releasing you from its hold.

Then, once you are satisfied that you have brought into this room everybody whom you associate with sorrow, grief and pain, take a deep breath and with a loud, expressive sigh, see each and every one of them being blown out of the room and far away into the universe by the force of this sigh. And, if you feel reluctant to let them go, understand that it is only the sorrow associated with their memory that you are releasing, not the happy moments you spent together.

So, finally, you are in this room of sorrow by yourself once more, and as you stand in the centre of this room, you reclaim your power and say out loud: 'I now leave sorrow and pain behind and understand that these need never enter into my life again. I am at peace within myself and am worthy of a life filled with happiness and joy.'

And then, you leave this room, closing the door behind you.

You then walk a little further down the corridor and come to a door behind which you feel a sparkling energy of lightness and fun. You see above the door the words: JOY, LAUGHTER, SATISFACTION.

You eagerly open the door and there in the centre of the room is an image of you as a child laughing and giggling and emitting a wonderful energy of lightness. And then, it is up to you to bring into this room all the people in your life you associate with times of joy, from your early childhood to the present time. And each person who comes in gives you a big, loving hug and with each new person, the atmosphere becomes more light and bouncy. If anyone comes into the room with a solemn expression, just ask them if they are in the right room and give them a kick up the ass!

Stay within this room as long as you like feeling the energy of love and joy fill your whole being, feeling its warmth, knowing that this is your birthright, that you can create this feeling in your life in the present and well into the future. Also, feel the energy within this room run through your veins healing your body and mind.

Finally, in your own time, take your leave from this room but carry with you that feeling of lightness, knowing that you can return there any time you want.

And then, walk back along and out of the corridor, slowly return to your body, and open your eyes.

Bereavement

Probably the most extreme case of sorrow and grief with relation to AIDS is that of someone whose lover or partner has died of the disease or, indeed, of any disease. There is an established link between bereavement and cancer, and, of course, the basic imbalance that allows AIDS to take hold within the body is exactly the same process by which cancer also attacks a person's system.

Not only does the lover of someone who dies of AIDS often have the long-lasting stress of looking after his or her partner, followed by the grief of the loss, the emptiness after so much sharing and even a vague sense of guilt of not having been able to do enough; but there is also the additional fear that he or she will come down with the disease.

Needless to say, it is necessary for anyone who has undergone such an ordeal to go through a period of grief and the most important thing to do is express this grief, whether through tears or words with friends or even in silent communion with that spiritual part of yourself in a quiet place or writing your feelings down. The important word, though, is expression. I have already explained what stoically keeping the pain within does to the body.

I have come across many instances of people whose experience of their lover dying has been a tremendous growing experience rather than just one of sadness. On one occasion, I had a long talk with a man who had lost his lover and the energy that emanated from him was astonishing. He told me how the first three months after his lover's diagnosis had been full of pain and anger, but finally this had brought the two of them even closer together with an unspoken intimacy and understanding that grew deeper as the months went by, even as it became apparent that his lover was going to die. The peace within his lover during those last weeks, when he had put all that was filled with sadness behind him, would remain with him forever, he said. It was this which had carried him through his period of mourning and he felt a greater strength and peace within himself to do what was really important to him for the rest of his life.

Of course, not everyone will have had it so 'easy' – the death of a loved one, especially of one so comparatively young, is probably the greatest hardship most of us will have to bear in our lives. Yet, even this – in particular this – is an experience that draws us deep within ourselves and makes us confront that age-old question of what life really means to us. It was, indeed, a similar experience which started me on the path which led me to write this book.

The spirit of one's lover can always remain with you, but the grief and sorrow, however deeply felt, must in time be released and left behind. The one thing that a confrontation with death, the finiteness of our earthly existence does is to bring us all closer to our true essence and to make us understand that there is no longer any point in putting up with any bullshit in life, the pretence, the need to conform. What is the point of going through all this suffering if we do not grow from it, become stronger and recognize that the limited span of our life is meant to be lived to the full, with our intuition and conscience as our only guide?

Fear

Fear is the very antithesis of feeling your own strength, that source of the Healer Within, because if you fear something, you immediately give it power over you.

This is how epidemics gain such momentum, whether it is 'flu, the bubonic plague or AIDS. Of course, there is the physical virus in the first place, but once a virus is seen as all-pervading, then the spectre of this tiny virus becomes lodged in people's minds as a threat of immense proportions. Take a minor disease like 'flu for example. How many times have you heard people say: 'I always seem to get 'flu at this time of the year' or 'Have you heard? There's a new strain of 'flu virus around'? Words, as I shall demonstrate later, are powerful things – in putting such thoughts into words, or even harbouring suppressed fear that such thoughts engender, you are putting energy into that entity we call 'flu or AIDS. Even by giving it a name, we give it an identity, a power of its own.

This may run counter to the rational way in which you have been taught cause and effect, but just think back on your life how fears have often become reality. Fear is an intangible force which governs the lives of so many people.

Fear manifests itself in many ways and is essentially a product of the rational mind. The one thing that I will always tell people, whether healthy or sick, is to learn to distinguish that inner voice of true intuition from the voice of fear – over the next few weeks, just try this out.

Throughout our lives, we are confronted with many choices, some minor, some major, and it is through the way we make these choices that we determine the direction of our lives: the ease or pain of our lives depends on these choices.

Sometimes, these present themselves as a clear cut decision between two opposites, yet, just as frequent, but less recognized, are those little flashes of inspiration that come through our mind just to do something because it feels right. And how often we dismiss such thoughts from our mind, because they are just 'too unconventional' or because the risks of following such a path seem too great.

This is why I say that fear is a product of the rational mind. Our intuition is that part of us which is in touch with the whole picture, whilst our rational mind is what divides everything into little parcels, separating this aspect of life from that. Our rational mind will always see reasons why we should not do things: i.e. the risks are too great; what other people will think; things are bad, but better the devil you know than the devil you don't know – and then, before you know it, fear sets in, paralyzes you and your intuitive feeling is swamped.

What has all this got to do with AIDS? you may ask.

In letting fear smother your intuition, you are turning away from your true self, your highest creativity. In the end, it is the law of the Universe that something will stop you short and make you think and learn and understand how you are running away from your essence. And, for many of us, that something is AIDS. And the way in which we confront this challenge is a symbol of the way we confront our selves. If we learn and follow our intuition and leave our fear and the past behind, focusing on our present being and true potential, then we can also leave AIDS behind.

If you fear something, this means you do not understand the metaphysical truth behind it. If something is blocking your way, it is there for a reason. If you fear it, you give it power over you; if you are willing to learn from it and understand why it is blocking your way, it will eventually dissolve.

How often in the past have I banged my head against an obstacle in my life when all it needed for it to disappear was for it to teach me a simple lesson. Nowadays, it is the common cold which always gives me the message that I am allowing something to have power over me because I am acting through fear or am not trusting my own intuition. I get a cold, which will stay with me until I recognize and let go of what I am allowing to obstruct my path; when I do let go, the cold and the obstacle disappear simultaneously and almost instantly.

AIDS is an infinitely more powerful message. Yet, if you go deep within yourself and peel away all those layers of fear, pain and of surrendering your own power, it is an even more powerful vehicle for change. When you have reached that essence within, that trust in yourself, then the balance within you will be naturally restored and your body will quite simply take care of itself.

To understand this means you must listen to your intuition and feel what is right. To put it into effect needs patience, for patience is trusting that something will happen in its own time; impatience, looking for an instant cure, is fearing deep down that it will not happen.

Fear of Intimacy

One of the most common fears that I find in people with AIDS is the fear of intimacy, something I touched on in the chapter on isolation.

Fear of intimacy is in reality a combination of many fears: it is the fear of being let down, hurt or rejected or making a fool of yourself; it is a lack of self-confidence; it is fear of opening up to another person the parts of yourself you have buried deepest, as this also means that you have to confront them yourself; it is fear of showing your own vulnerability, even the fear of showing parts of yourself of which you are secretly ashamed. But, the root of it all is simply the fear of letting go, following your intuition and putting your trust in another person.

And the reasons behind this fear are just as diverse: there

may have been a particularly bad experience in the past upon which you judge other people; a parent or a person of authority may have told you never to trust anyone or that you should always keep a part of you secret; within men in particular, there is the ridiculous social pressure of equating 'masculinity' with not showing your feelings. The list is endless . . . and sad.

For intimacy is the truest expression of your highest self, of that loving part of you. It is also the essence of balance: of giving and receiving equally.

And once more, the only guide to the degree you open up to another person is your intuition. Everybody has that gut feeling – not to be confused with a sexual feeling! – when we meet someone with whom we feel particularly comfortable and in tune, yet how many of us have the courage to follow this up and allow a relationship, at whatever level, to develop in its own way.

And, when I talk about intimacy, I do not mean the tendancy of certain people to be open and smiling and friendly to everyone they meet, yet beneath this superficial geniality, the barriers to true intimacy are even thicker. You can fool others but, in the end, you cannot fool your body. Be honest with yourself and be aware of the depth of intimacy to which you are prepared to go.

For this is the message I wish to get over, as I shall more forcibly in the chapter on love. Only if you are able to open your heart and truly express your inner self will the Healer Within be fully activated; if you turn away from this, you turn away from your source of inner strength.

Which brings me to one final, very specific fear.

The Fear of Getting Well

Your first reaction to seeing this heading may well be: 'How sick! How can anyone be afraid of getting better?'

My answer to that is this: think back to what I have already written about the emptiness within a person giving space for the AIDS consciousness to enter into them and you may begin to see a stumbling block that may confront certain

PWAs – even those who have reacted to their diagnosis in an ultimately positive manner.

For not an inconsiderable amount of people, AIDS has proven to be the gigantic kick up the ass that I have mentioned. In being confronted with their own mortality, with the 'challenge of AIDS', they have seen the potential for growth and change within themselves and others. This has often taken the form of forming support groups with other PWAs, going out speaking to outside organizations about coping with the disease and, in particular, finding a new sense of community and belonging directly as a result of being a person with AIDS.

Yet, sometimes, lurking in the deep recesses of their mind is the question: 'If I attain the ultimate goal and rid myself of this disease, will I then not return to the emptiness and lack of purpose that was in my life before I got sick?' Sounds an unlikely question, but it is not uncommon.

It is a very easy mistake to make, associating the growth that one has undergone with the disease of AIDS itself, as opposed to seeing that AIDS was purely a means of initiating that growth. Instead of appreciating that they themselves have directed their own growth within and that this growth will continue, they see it as beginning and ending with AIDS.

So, when I write about the fear of getting well, I really mean the fear of returning to the past, but, of course, no one ever returns to the past after such a period of intense change unless they make a very conscious decision to do so.

Indeed, this particular fear shows what lies at the very heart of the emotion of fear: a sense of one's own limitation – i.e. 'I've remained healthy for so long, but I can't fully cure myself.' This is why it is so important to understand one's own creativity.

Creativity and Limitation

So, what do I really mean by creativity? To most people, the word conjures up the image of some artistic talent, which is indeed part of it. Yet, creativity is something much broader than this. It is, as the word says, the ability to create one's own reality – *from within.*

What is the essence of creativity in an artistic sense? Quite simply, it is, to begin with, recognizing a particular ability and then giving it free expression. How many of us see great actors, musicians, painters etc. and wish we had their talent, or, more to the point, wish we had a particular talent through which we could express that inner part of ourselves?

The truth is, of course, that we all have an incredible well of creativity within us – every single one of you reading this book. It may not be something that leads to fame, such as the talents mentioned above, – and who needs fame anyway? – but we all have something within us that is special to ourselves, which is there just waiting to be released and freely expressed. It may be as a carpenter, a designer, a gardener or a technician; it may be as a teacher, an adviser and comforter of other people, a special knack with children or the elderly – the diversity of man is infinite.

For many of us, it takes a long time for us to recognize where this special creativity within us truly lies. From early childhood, we are constantly bombarded by those things we 'ought' to do through the expectations of our parents and family, but this more often than not has more to do with conformity and earning a living than true creativity. And, of course, as we grow older, most of us bend to the will and collective pressure of the so-called 'standards' of society.

It often takes a major upset in our lives for us to really confront and accept our true creativity. How many of us have settled into a comfortable routine existence, accepting second best, instead of actively going out and fulfilling that creative side of us?

Well, AIDS, whether the reality or the fear of it, can be the most gigantic vehicle to unleash that creativity within you. It has brought you to a stop to face yourself – not the picture you offer to the world, not just the parts of you that you choose to acknowledge, not just you as a career person, a lover, a parent, but as a whole, complete being. And, within that whole, is your very essence, the true expression of your very individual self.

MEDITATION NO. 6

As before, you centre yourself and enter into the corridor which is your second chakra. You walk to the end of the corridor into a room marked CREATIVITY.

As you shut the door behind you and turn to the centre of the room, you create in front of you an image of yourself in whatever you feel to be your most creative guise, whether as a teacher, actor, carpenter, counsellor etc., even as a parent or a lover. As you do so, you become that figure and feel what it is like inside you when you express that creative part of you.

Then, as you are expressing this creative instinct within you – and it does not have to be just one – somebody out of your past comes up and tells you that you are actually not creative in this way. This opens the floodgates and, one by one, all those people who have tried to turn you away from your creativity and have tried to impose limitation upon you come up to you.

As each one comes before you and you listen to their judgment of you, you take them by the hand and say: 'I thank you for your opinion of me and what you think is right for me. However, this is only your view of me, of what perhaps you want me to be. It has nothing to do with who I really am.' You release them, let them stand to one side and allow the next to come before you: parents who wanted something for you which was not really you; teachers who said you were not good enough; peers who dismissed your idea of creativity as inferior to theirs; the countless people who have tried to impose their limited vision of reality upon you.

Finally, you bring in front of yourself that figure which is you, for you have surely at times during your life put limitations on your creativity, saying: 'Oh no! I'm not capable of that!' And, just as with all the others, you take this figure by the hand and release it too.

When you have done this, you line up all these people, and you blow a whistle. From the depths of the room, a train comes chugging in – it is marked: *Expresstrain to Limitation*. All these people climb on board, you give another whistle and the train chugs out of the room, into the corridor and out into the distance. So, now, you are left alone in this room and within this new space, you can create your own reality. You affirm and see in this room the reality you wish to create – not just the outward trappings of your creative guise, but your ability to bring into your life what you want and know you deserve, from health and fitness to warm relationships and prosperity.

Finally, when you are satisfied that you have covered all you need to, you leave this room of creativity, knowing that this is your birthright and you return to your body.

The Third Chakra: Power and Strength

As I mentioned at the beginning of the book, the connection between AIDS and the whole concept of power and strength may seem obscure to say the least. Indeed, when I first started healing through the chakras, the third always seemed to be the most obscure and certainly the least relevant to health and disease.

How wrong I was!

In fact, it has so much to do with the imbalance which allows AIDS into our system that, each time I have worked individually with a person with AIDS, I have learnt another lesson about this 'energy centre', for it is here that the greatest blockage occurs within virtually every person with AIDS I have dealt with.

So, what do these two rather nebulous words, power and strength, really mean and what relevance do they have to our health and the balance within our bodies?

Let me start with power and the two ends of the spectrum which are relevant here.

On the one hand, there is the way in which we all to varying degrees put out our power, using control, manipulation, possessiveness, judgment etc. as an integral part of our life.

On the other side of the coin, there is the way in which we relinquish the power we have over our own lives and submit to the views and actions of others.

These two supposed opposites are by no means mutually exclusive. As I will show you in an example later on, the one can actually feed the other, continuously jumping backwards and forwards from one end of the spectrum to the other.

And, in between those two extremes of power is Strength. Strength is the very central core of our being, that inner part of us which is essentially the starting point of the Healer Within.

As you have by now noted, much of all this overlaps with what I have already written concerning the second chakra, and, indeed, the second and third chakras are inextricably linked. Although the second is the seat of our emotional development, it is the way in which we control and suppress our emotions that allows them to assume power over us.

In this section, I shall not be dealing with specific emotions and the hold we allow them to have over us. Instead, I shall be concentrating on the deeper, more fundamental way in which we allow that inner strength within us to be sucked out of us and how, most often quite subconsciously, we draw our own energy from ourselves and invest it in thoughts and actions which ultimately give us nothing in return.

Control

When I mentioned power just now, I referred to the two supposed ends of the spectrum: putting one's power out in terms of control and manipulation, and giving up one's own power by allowing oneself to be controlled. In reality, the one has a great deal to do with the other, and this inter-relationship, this swinging between the one and the other, is very important when we are looking at the imbalance within a person with AIDS.

Let me illustrate this with an example of a person with AIDS, whom I shall call John.

I went to see John at the request of a friend of his. John had had AIDS for just over a year and his body was covered literally head to toe with KS lesions.

Before becoming sick, his was outwardly the perfect existence. He had a very successful, albeit high-pressured career, which earned him a lot of money. He had a beautiful apartment, travelled a lot between America and Europe, was considered very attractive, easy going, with lots of friends and seemingly no problems whatsoever. On the surface, he had the ideal existence.

Yet, when I went to see him, the dead weight that I felt emanating from the area of his third chakra was heavier than anything I had ever felt before.

The story behind it all was this.

John's father had been, until his retirement, an extremely

successful, aggressive, self-made businessman. Although, as he grew up, John was emotionally closer to his mother, there was the continuing pressure from his father, often unspoken, to go out and make a career for himself. Without really taking into account what his son wanted, the father made certain openings for him which would allow him to start on the path towards success. Sure enough, driven by the desire to prove himself coupled with an innate intelligence, John became successful very quickly. The fact that he had wanted to go to university and have a spell of freedom rather than embark on a career straight from school was soon forgotten.

That was the first stage. Having reached this level of success, where did he go from there? From time to time, he would wonder where it all led and what the point of it all was, but such doubts were soon swept under the carpet. He had thought how nice it would be to take a year off, but the figure of his father still loomed in the background.

As time went by, he developed a great social life, lots of acquaintances, wild parties and the drugs that went with them. He had no problem meeting people for sex, but, as far as relationships were concerned, he always seemed to end up with people who were rather domineering and were incapable of showing any warmth: almost a reflection of his outer self. His friends were not the kind of people he could relate too deeply to; they tended to be drawn to the image of perfect control which he projected, and, in the end, he grew to like the idea of having this 'circle' around him.

So, with all of this going for him, why did he end up getting sick? It has all to do with Control.

From the very instant that he made the decision to follow his father's vision of him rather than his own, he started on a merry-go-round which became faster and faster and increasingly more difficult to get off. From the feeling of having to prove himself and get approval from others, of always having to do better, came that drive to control every aspect of his life, to structure and plan his existence around a goal that he did not fully understand. When he was away from this treadmill, he reckoned he deserved the pleasure of going to the other extreme of going wild and losing control. And, as he became more and more an image of success in other people's eyes, he gradually came to see his life through their eyes. Every so often, deep down, he would feel an inner yearning for something simpler and more meaningful, but, by then, he could not let the mask of control fall.

For that is what it had become: a mask of control. He always had to maintain an image, the hard shell over a void of emptiness, the need to control for fear of losing control. During the day, he was the model of self-control, the successful businessman, being able to handle and manipulate any situation; during the night, the pent-up tension was released in a frenzy of constant activity.

In relationships, the reason he always attracted the same kind of person was that this seemed the one way to relinquish this control. In the quiet of a 'private' life, he wanted the very opposite of his 'public' life – he wanted someone to take over control, but constantly confused the giving and receiving of a warm, loving relationship with the projection he made of someone who would be dominant and take any responsibility of the relationship away from him. He was often left hurt and with the feeling of being used by such people.

When I first went to see him, he was polite, but saw my visit as an intrusion (which is why I almost never see people unless they come to me). I worked on him once and then, when I was working with him during my second visit, there was a reaction like an exploding gun, an anger directed towards me with a vehemence I had never before experienced: what had I done to deserve to be so healthy, when he who had done no wrong was sick? It all poured out and eventually turned to tears; he finally expressed his true feelings of sadness because people had never really loved him for who he was, and of fear that, if he did get better, he would return to that sense of emptiness that had gnawed away inside him for years before.

In the end, he did die, but only after he had found a certain peace within himself, making peace with and expressing his feelings to his family and friends. He died because, deep down, he made the choice, believing that this was the only way not to have to struggle any more. I respect his choice, although dying is by no means the only way to rise above having to struggle and keep a controlling grip on life.

I have spent so long describing this somewhat extreme case, because there are elements within this story which apply in varying degrees to the majority of the cases of AIDS I have encountered.

The essence of this story is: *not being true to oneself.*

This can be manifested in so many ways: being constantly influenced and worried by other people's opinions or making decisions because they follow the route of conformity rather than an individual gut feeling are but a couple of examples. Fundamentally, it is a matter of consciously or subconsciously giving up your power to other people or to outside forces.

At the beginning, it is a process that can easily be reversed, but, as time goes by, such behaviour can become so ingrained that one's true desires and creativity become relegated to the deep recesses of the subconscious. The gulf between one's inner aspirations and the outer mask is not just symbolic; as this gulf becomes wider, a very real and ever growing emptiness develops between them, a void which allows a consciousness such as AIDS to enter within. And, to make matters worse, those who have developed this mask are the first to fool themselves and others into believing that there is nothing lacking inside. I have lost count of those who have angrily denied any such lack when I have first pointed it out to them, only for them to admit to it later on.

It all goes back to the chapter on creativity. When we ignore our true creativity, our inner selves, we are literally turning our backs on ourselves, our inner strength. This leads in turn to a suppression of other aspects of our lives – our emotions, our true feelings and aspirations – until a lingering sense of dissatisfaction and lack of fulfilment becomes almost accepted as something which must be born in life: the philosophy of 'You can't have your cake and eat it.'

In the case I have just illustrated, a seemingly ideal

existence concealed a deep-felt emptiness, and the control needed to hide this void from other people literally tore his mind and body apart. His was certainly the most extreme case of this that I have encountered, yet it would do no harm for all of us to look closely at ourselves and see to what extent we have surrendered our power to others and buried our true selves and aspirations under the superficial goals which our society rates so highly.

MEDITATION NO. 7

As with the previous few meditations, you centre yourself, come out of your body and, this time, face your third chakra at your solar plexus. Again, you see a corridor stretch out in front of you and you walk along this until you come to a door marked AUTHORITY FIGURES.

As you walk into the room behind the door, you prepare yourself to bring in front of you all those people and entities that you have at some point in your life allowed to have power over you.

First of all, you bring in front of you your parents. They appear before you, you take them both by the hand, and, as you do so, the image of them is transformed. Suddenly, they are standing in front of you, completely naked and alone. You see them for what they are – two people whose lives, like yours, have been a succession of experiences, good and bad, and who are just what they are. They are neither perfect nor totally bad. They just are, and, as you see them naked in front of you, you know that they can have no power over you. For once and for all, you release any sense that you must live your life according to their values.

Likewise, you bring into your presence any other members of your family and have them stand naked in front of you, releasing any hold they have over you.

Then, you bring into your presence other stereotypic-al authority figures, such as teachers, priests, and, in particular, doctors. And they stand before you, naked and alone, human beings like yourself with their own ups and downs in their personal lives. Their views may be right for their own lives, but have no hold over yours. As your doctors stand there, naked, in front of you, telling you that you will be lucky to live more than two years and the best you can hope for is to be on this or that drug, you know that they are passing on to you their limited view of reality and that their pronounce-ments have no power over you.

Then, you bring into your presence all those at work or in other spheres of your life who seem to have some measure of control over your life, and you take them by the hand and their clothes just fall off them, leaving these naked figures in front of you, which can have no power over you. You do not judge them; you accept them as they are and let them go.

Next, you bring before you all those people you consider to be more powerful than you – people who seem to be more successful, more attractive, whose lives seem to be easier or more exciting, everybody you look up to. Again, you take them by the hand and they appear naked in front of you, neither greater nor smaller than you, and you realize that comparison is worthless. They are what they are; you are what you are, no less creative than them, only creative in your own individual way.

Once you have gone through all individuals you know who have exerted some power over you, you turn to other symbols of authority. You bring before you a certain type of person you try and emulate, or the symbol of the kind of society you have felt you must conform to. When you take them by the hand, they too stand naked and helpless in front of you, neither more nor less powerful than you – just different.

Likewise, you bring forward those people or symbols who have judged you for what you are and, as they stand naked before you, you see that they have no power, let alone right, to impose their personal views upon you.

Moving forward even from symbols, you visualize objects, entities or abstract ideas which you have allowed to hold sway over you.

First, you see AIDS in front of you and see it as a microscopic virus. You put out your hand to touch it, and, as you do so, it disintegrates. You reclaim your power and know that no such tiny organism can have power over you.

In the same way, you see drugs or alcohol or any other substance which you have allowed to have power over you. You put out your hand to touch them and see them disintegrate before your eyes. And you understand that you do not need them any longer.

Then, you bring into your presence anything that seems to stand in your way. If you are always short of money, you see a pile of bills in front of you; you reach out and touch them and they too disintegrate, so that you know that they too have no power over you and that you can create your own material prosperity. And you do likewise with anything else that blocks your way. You put your hand out with faith and see it disintegrate as it has no power over you.

Finally, you stand in this room and look around at all the naked figures surrounding you. You see that not one of them has any kind of authority over you; as you look at them, naked, exactly as they are, you take a deep breath and reclaim mastery over your own life, responsibility from your own decisions and actions.

Then, in your own time, you leave this room, walk out of your third chakra and back into your body.

Power and Addiction

The most obvious manifestation of letting outside forces have power over you is addictive behaviour. Of course, most people tend to think of drug addiction or alcoholism, but addictions go far beyond this to include sex, work, status, even compulsive buying of clothes. There are not too many people who have no form of addiction whatsoever in their lives.

So, what is addiction? It is, on the one hand, letting something have power over you, an obsession. But, on a deeper and much more important level, addiction is the need to fill the void inside you.

As AIDS is very much associated with the addictive intake of drugs, I wish to spend a little time on this – not on the obvious fact that shared needles are a principal way of passing on the virus, not on the equally self-evident fact that an excess of drugs, even antibiotics, causes havoc to the physical balance within our bodies, but on the fundamental root cause of addiction and how an understanding of it can help to break the cycle.

As someone who has tried a few of the the 'lighter' recreational drugs, I find it very easy to see how any drug can become addictive, for, like no other substance, do they take you on a high far away from 'reality'. They seem to be quite simply a wonderful temporary escape from day to day existence. And, needless to say, when people start taking them, they never think in terms of addiction.

But, for many people, these short term escapes into a realm of no cares begin to appear to be the only way out from the 'sordid reality' and drudgery of their day to day existence. From that point on, addiction is assured: there is the agonizing depression of coming down from a high, which makes 'reality' seem worse and worse and the desire to escape it stronger and stronger.

You will note that the word 'reality' keeps popping up again and again, and this is in many ways the key to the state of mind which allows addictive behaviour to take hold. If we perceive the so-called real world as unjust or superficial and we feel out of tune with it, that same old feeling of isolation and emptiness starts creeping back into the picture again.

I know only too well from my own experience the confusion that can be felt when confronted by a society which seems to be obsessed with superficial and material things with no apparent concern for the more human, personal aspects of life. Yet, even if this reality seems to be unbearable and you try to escape it through drugs or whatever means, you are adding to the power of this 'real' world. You are quite simply saying: 'I do not like it. I can do nothing about it, so I will escape it as much as I can' – yet another example of turning away from your own strength and yielding power to the source of your discontent.

What increases the sense of isolation is the scorn which this same society heaps upon people who become addicted to drugs. It is the beginning of a vicious circle. First, the escape from a society whose values mean nothing to you, followed by the judgment of that society and increasingly compounded by a feeling of lack of self-worth.

Each of these stages on the downward spiral are tantamount to giving up your own source of inner strength, first by running away from the world and yourself and then by seeing yourself as others see you, accepting that you do not deserve the best in your life. And, the more you surround yourself with other people who share this low view of themselves, the more this feeling of powerlessness will feed itself.

If your life seems full of hardship and you are constantly condemning the world as being unjust to you, then you are seeing yourself as a mere pawn in the game of life rather than drawing upon that inner reserve of energy to direct your own life. If, on the other hand, you confront this seeming injustice and understand that the only reality that faces you is the one you create, you can start to see yourself as you are: an individual in your own right who can build your own life on that nature within you which is special to you.

In a strange way, to admit that you are special needs courage, as this means accepting that you are responsible for creating your own destiny rather than seeing your life as being at the mercy of outside forces. It also means breaking that vicious circle created by judgment, both by and of others and of oneself.

Judgment, Ego and Comparison

Just think how many times in a day you judge other people, even your closest friends, and, of course, yourself. Judgment is all to do with power and comparison, nothing to do with inner strength.

In the case of self-judgment, it is again a matter of surrendering your own power. How many of us feel that we are not physically attractive, not too bright or amusing or interesting, and how often do we allow this to filter down to a deeper judgment of ourselves and see ourselves as inferior beings compared with other people around us? It is this self-judgment which robs us of the feeling of our own self-worth and this ultimately leads us to believe that we have no power to create what we really want in our lives.

Judgment is an extension of ego, which is at the very centre of the third chakra and is the antithesis of inner strength. Ego is that part of us which must always see ourselves in comparison with other people and which constantly plays games, sometimes putting us on a pedestal, sometimes putting us down. There is no harmony and strength within ego because it is always rushing from one extreme to another, putting energy out towards things that have little to do with our essential being.

Ego is need – the need always to be searching for something to attach ourselves to. It is that compulsive desire to see things and in particular people in relation to ourselves rather than as entities in their own right. Material ambition and competition are each forms of this need, just as jealousy and envy are results of this mentality. Instead of being at peace with ourselves, there is the constant need to compare our state of being with others, as if this were the only way of judging our own self-worth.

The more we build up expectations of ourselves and of other people, the more we judge when these expectations are not met. As soon as we build up an expectation of somebody, we are putting them into a strait-jacket of our own making – we are basically seeing this person as a projection of ourselves rather than as the individual that he or she is.

This is what possessiveness is all about. If you are in a relationship and are inclined to be in the least bit possessive, whether as a lover, parent or friend, what is really going on? You are holding on to the person in question because you are afraid that you will lose this person. In holding on to someone, you are giving into fear and, in doing so, your ego is trying to control this person, rather than letting the person have his or her freedom. If two people are going to be together in a relationship, this will be so because they both choose freely to be together – if one person tries to control and smother another, the natural flow between them is destroyed and the relationship will ultimately die. Possessiveness is the very opposite of trust, and no relationship can survive without trust.

This is so important to understand, as I have seen many people with AIDS who have been through the harrowing experience of vainly holding on to someone in a relationship way past the time the energy has faded between the two partners. It is of course not easy to let go of someone and face the prospect of being alone, even though you know that the relationship has come to an end; yet the internal damage is even greater if you continue to put your own energy and source of strength out to someone who will give you nothing in return.

Likewise, on a very different level, lust is an extension of ego. When we lust after somebody or something, we are simply wanting to possess them. This lies at the root of promiscuity – if we see someone we find attractive, we are, by wanting to have sex with them, wanting to possess that beauty, even for a little while. If it is purely for the sensual fulfilment, we are treating the person in question as an extension of our own desire.

Why is it that I am focusing so much on ego and judgment and what does this all have to do with health, balance and AIDS?

First of all, all activity of the ego, from possessiveness to judgment, from competitiveness to an inferiority complex, means that you are putting your energy out in a totally uncreative sense. It means that you are trying to control and make everything into a struggle rather than letting your intuition guide you in all the major decisions of your life. There is an inner tension and stress behind all behaviour related to the ego – remember what I wrote about the relationship between the third chakra and the adrenal glands in the opening part of this book.

Secondly, your ego draws you away from truly relating to other people. The act of judgment, for instance, is basically an act of intolerance. It gives power to that part of you which says that what is right for you is right for everybody, rather than understanding that everyone has the right to act in their own way and create their own reality.

Indeed, judgment betrays an inability to see deep within yourself as much as an unwillingness to relate deeply to others. Just for a moment think of the person you judge most, who irritates you most. Then, think of what it is about this person which you judge most of all and try to understand how this relates to you. The reason I ask you to do this is that, when we judge a particular aspect of another person's character or behaviour, it is because this is a reflection of an aspect within our own character or behaviour that we like least of all. When I was first told this, my first reaction was one of ridicule, but, once I was honest with myself and looked really deeply at my own behaviour, I understood how very true this was.

Judgment, possessiveness, competitiveness, lust, jealousy and much more – all are aspects of ego. Each time we behave and react in this way, we are viewing another person as an extension of ourselves and we are therefore not relating to them as individuals in their own right. Our ego, the focal point of imbalance within this third chakra, is the very antithesis of love, and in being so, draws us away from that highest healing element within us.

Strength and Faith

Compared with the constant activity of the ego, inner strength may seem somewhat boring, but, in reality, it is quite the opposite, as it opens one up to the endless possibilities of one's own creativity.

Just think back over your life and remember those few people you have encountered who radiate a wonderful sense of stillness and inner peace, for whom life appears to be so simple. They may not at first sight be the most lively and exciting people, but they give off an aura of quiet strength and trust which most of us would like to feel within ourselves.

Inner strength has nothing to do with power and ego. It just is. Inner strength is based on faith – it does not need to compare, because it knows that intuition and knowledge within are the only guides.

I touched briefly on faith at the beginning of this book, but it is now time for me to explain what I really mean by this word.

Faith in the traditional religious sense means a belief in an all powerful God which is completely separate from us, ruling and dispensing justice from above. Traditional religion has come to be shrouded in dogma, rules and, more often than not, intolerance. In many cases, it puts more emphasis on the concept of sin and evil, rather than on good. It has also, over the years, been used as a tool for power, for manipulation of the masses.

The faith which I talk about has little to do with this. There are no set rules, no judgment. Faith is purely an understanding of the source of one's own strength.

The Universe is a seemingly limitless space around us – even our magnificent Solar System is just a drop in the ocean of this space. Yet, within this immeasurable entity, there is one very simple law: every form of life is interdependent. On a simple level, you just have to look at what we call Nature and see how, in a certain environment, all living creatures have between them a cycle of interdependence which enables them to survive.

What man has over the years tried to conceptualize as God is neither just a vague concept, nor some old man sitting in his celestial palace. God is that Whole which we call the Universe, the Energy which links everything together. We are all an integral part of this Whole, and each of us is, within this, an individual being with our own special nature.

The essential work of the ego is to make us see our separateness, as opposed to our connection with this limitless Universe. It makes us see our achievements as arising solely from our own intellect and power; it tells us that we are alone in the world and must struggle for ourselves without expecting any help from outside – and when things go wrong, it is just cruel fate or chance. The ego sees faith as blind passivity, a substitute for those who are not bright or 'privileged' enough to think and act for themselves.

That ego part of us does not recognize that thinking, acting and individuality are all essential to faith and inner strength.

The fact that we are all connected to that ultimate source of energy – the Universe, God, whatever you like to call it – does not mean that we immediately must surrender our individuality and become part of an amorphous mass. Nor does it mean that we have no responsibility and no power over our destiny. What it does mean is that we can tap into this source of limitless energy and potential and draw from it whenever we wish.

From the moment we are born, we are bombarded by a

whole host of influences and patterns which mould us into the individual beings which we become. Unless we choose to surround ourselves with rigidity, this individuality is constantly changing as we perceive and continue to absorb all that happens around us.

As we grow older, we are confronted by more and more choices and possibilities. Every day, we have to make lots of minor decisions, but it is the major choices which determine the direction of our lives. We are only rarely confronted with these, but they invariably come at such particularly crucial points in our lives that we must always be open to act on and not walk away from such choices. The way we react to AIDS is such a choice – on the level not only of physical health, but also of the way we take responsibility for the rest of our lives.

This is the essence of faith: knowing that we have the responsibility for the direction of our lives in our own hands and understanding that the path will be full of peace and joy if only we follow our intuition, our true nature. There is no such thing as blind fate. In a Universe where everything is interrelated, what we call chance or fate is in reality the myriad of connections which we have to that limitless energy within the Universe. If we follow our intuition, we know when and how we can draw upon this energy.

It is only our ego which tells us otherwise. Our ego piles layer upon layer over this intuitive sense – as we get swept away following goals and behaving in a way that has little to do with our true nature and aspirations, we lose our intuitive connection with that Universal Energy. The road towards regaining that connection is by necessity one of patience, gradually peeling off layer after layer, letting go of all the excess baggage that you do not wish to carry with you into the future, until you reach that inner core of yourself. AIDS is merely a stimulus for this change, and, like the rest of this excess, can also be left behind once this function is fulfilled.

MEDITATION NO. 8

Once again, centre yourself, come out of your body and walk into this corridor which is your third chakra. As you walk along, you see on the walls seven barometers, each of them graded on a scale of zero to one hundred.

You walk up to the first one and you see the word POWER inscribed on it. As you stand before it, you look at your life and see how much you use power in your day to day dealings with people. How much do you manipulate and play games with other people? How possessive or jealous are you? How competitive or how ambitious for recognition and material goals are you? How rigidly do you try to control, structure and plan your life, rather than just following your intuition? How much do you judge others and, above all, yourself? On a scale of zero to one hundred, how do you think you rate in the power game? If you rate higher than you truly wish, then know that you can come back any time and see this barometer fall, by letting go of the *need* to continuously put out power and control.

You then leave this behind and walk up to the next barometer which is marked STRENGTH. How much of life is based on inner strength rather than power? How much do you follow your inner voice rather than the opinions of others and of society? How much peace do you feel within yourself, rather than the need to be constantly going out and doing things? How much confidence do you have in your ability to create your own path in life, or do you still see yourself at the mercy of other people or of fate? From zero to one hundred, how strong are you within yourself?

The next barometer is COURAGE. How much do you stand up for what you feel is right, not just in the company of friends, but in all situations in your life? How much are you prepared to take your life by the scruff of its neck and follow your intuitive path, even if your rational side sees it as being too risky? How much are you prepared to run against the tide, be unconventional, as long as it feels right? How courageous are you, from zero to one hundred?

You then move on to COWARDICE. How often do you run away from things, especially your true self and the important choices you have to make? How often are you confronted with a choice and you take the easy option because it is less of a risk? How often do you shrink away from standing up for yourself or friends when you know that you or they are right? How much do you surrender your power to other people and live your life through their eyes rather than your own? How much do you surrender to fear? From zero to one hundred, how do you figure on the scale of cowardice?

The next barometer is HONESTY. How honest are you with other people? How truly do you express your emotions rather than bottling them up inside? How much do you hide from even your closest friends because you are ashamed of something in your life? And, just as important, how honest are you with yourself? How much do you play games with yourself, suppressing within you things that are important?

You then move on to TRUST. How much do you trust other people, or, more to the point, how much do you trust your intuitive feel for other people? How prepared are you to open yourself up to other people on a deep and meaningful level? Most important of all, how much do you trust your intuition? If you feel it is right to do something, do you just go ahead and do it? How much trust do you have in yourself as a divine being who can follow that higher self within you and create your own reality? How much do you trust in that Universal Energy to provide for you if you are prepared to put out to it what you really want?

The final barometer is PROSPERITY. Prosperity does not just mean material prosperity; it means that you are worthy to have in your life anything that you feel is right. How worthy do you think you are of having the highest and the best in your life? Do you put limitations upon yourself? Do you believe that you will have the highest and best relationship, no financial problems, no need to struggle in your life? Do you believe that you deserve to be perfectly healthy and therefore will be so? From zero to one hundred, how high is your prosperity consciousness?

You now leave these barometers behind, knowing that, at any time, you can return to them and move them up and down as you wish, knowing that it is purely up to you at what level they remain.

You then walk along the corridor until, right at the end, you come to a door which bears the inscription: STRENGTH. As you approach it, the door swings open of its own accord and there in front of you, glowing with a bright light, is the archetypal symbol of the Sword. It is hanging there in thin air and you know it is there for you. Although it is almost your size, you take it by the hilt and, as you lift it up above your head, it feels so light, yet full of energy. You practise swinging it around you and you know that this is the sword of your inner strength that you can draw upon at any time to cut through intolerance, through doubt, to sweep away anything that stands in the path towards your highest good. It is there for you, for no one but you.

In your own time, you release this sword, once you feel comfortable with it, allowing it to hang there as it was before. You then turn and walk back towards the entrance to the corridor, knowing that you can return to pick up this sword of your own strength at any time.

Finally, you leave your third chakra behind, return to your own body and open your eyes.

3

The Healer Within

The Fourth Chakra: the Heart Centre

The fourth chakra, the heart centre, is often known as the 'Gateway to Heaven', because, in leaving the first three chakras behind, we are also leaving behind those aspects of ourselves which hold us back from our highest good. Only by understanding and letting go of all these outside forces which weigh us down can the true spirit within us rise up, grow and be freely expressed in our lives.

It has been necessary to painstakingly go through and identify all those 'lower' aspects of ourselves, for, if we still carry them on board, we cannot reach the higher elements within us – the strength and energy within is unable to be released to create the Healer Within.

For, remember, the heart centre is the seat of the thymus, the regulator of the immune system. If this centre is closed, so too is the thymus and the functioning of the immune system is impaired.

Throughout this book, I have been writing about our inner selves, the core of our existence and the deep sense of emptiness that many, consciously or subsconsciously, feel within. Yet, I have only fleetingly touched on how we can expand that core within us to fill that void, that emptiness within.

Well, this will be the focus of the rest of this book, so that you may get a feel of what is your true source of strength, that essence within you which creates the foundation from which to create your own reality and, among other things, to heal yourself.

In a word, you could describe this essence as love.

But, of course, a word is just a word and, for many, the word 'love' has very wishy-washy or, at the other end of the spectrum, too specific connotations. Nearly every song you hear on the radio is about love in one way or another; there is the state of being 'in love' – there are endless variations within the feelings associated with the word. You may say you love your parents, your spouse or lover, your friends, your children, but the way you feel towards each of them is different.

Therefore, leave behind any preconceptions you have about love; we are going to strip away from it all but the barest essentials. We shall see that Love, in its truest form, has no boundaries and is the *highest form of spirit* that we can attain in our earthly form.

Man is both a physical and spiritual being. We are all living creatures in a physical form: we need food and water to survive, we create attachments and possessions around us, we relate to each other in a physical sense. Within this physical form is our spiritual nature, that combination of intellect and intuition, where we look beyond the physical and feel things that cannot be explained in physical terms.

Love is the essence of our spiritual nature and also of our physical being, as it bridges the gap between the two and fuses them into one. It is an aspiration that all of us harbour deep within us, or, more to the point, it is *the* aspiration we all have deep within us, because it is through love that we come to realize and draw upon the deep connection we have with that Whole, which we call the Universe or God. Love is that central part of us, that core, which is our truest guide to our thoughts and actions: it is our conscience, and also, through the physical mechanism of the heart and the thymus, it is the pulse of our life and our protector.

Relationships

Strip away all possessions, all ambition etc., and what are we left with? Our fellow human beings.

We may of course get a temporary sense of pleasure or relief from the material things around us, but the essence of our lives is our relationship with our fellow human beings. It is through our contact with other people that we develop and grow, feel joy and pain. People are the hub and focus of our lives; it is the way in which we choose to relate to them that determines the course of our existence.

I say 'choose', as the way in which we choose to relate to people is the most important fundamental choice in our lives. It is a choice which has a bearing on every aspect of our existence, right down to the physical state of our bodies.

So, how do we define this choice?

I am going to illustrate this by concentrating on what comes first of all to people's minds when they talk about love: that relationship with a special partner. The way in which we handle this relationship is always a perfect reflection of the way in which we relate to people on a much broader scale, even of the way in which we relate to ourselves.

Let us briefly turn to the previous chapter on strength and power, for the barriers which our ego builds between ourselves and other people are what ultimately lead us away from a true understanding of love. For instance, when people talk or sing about love, they are most often referring to two people being 'in love', a state which has very little to do with love in its purest sense.

All of us have been through that state of being 'in love' with someone and many of us still strive to attain that supposed ideal. What this expression usually signifies, though, especially in the initial stages of instant attraction, is the process by which we project a fantasy or an image on to the other person – quite often, this image is a reflection of ourselves or of a particular need and we are indeed falling in love with this rather than the person in question.

This brings us to the question of expectation raised in the last chapter – it is a process of our ego and rational mind which divides people up into little parcels, expecting each tiny part to be just right, to fit into place like every piece of a jigsaw. As with all aspects of ego, this view of relationships leads to nothing but limitation. It destroys the infinite possibilities and natural flow that the variety of human relationships can afford us in our lives.

What is more, one cannot live in the state of being 'in love' forever – in day to day existence with a partner, a projected image cannot last, and, if it does, this means that there is no genuine trust and understanding between two people. Ultimately, the image will fall and, as the expectation is shattered, judgment will set in – the person holding on to the image will feel cheated, but, in reality, it is that person who has cheated him or herself.

This is just one of the choices we make when we view a relationship. Another relates to dependence.

Dependence, just like possessiveness, is another form of attachment and is related to this state of expectation and projection of an image. Of course, we all desire a mutually supportive relationship, but there are many who see this support as essential to their existence, where the projection they are imposing on their partner is that of someone stronger than themselves. Such projections have more to do with need than love.

Need and trust are opposites of each other in this respect.

A relationship where one partner needs the other in order to feel that he or she is a complete person inevitably puts pressure on the relationship by disturbing the natural balance between two individuals. In feeling a simple sense of trust, on the other hand, two partners acknowledge each other's rights as individuals and, most important of all, understand that each of them is fundamentally responsible for his or her own happiness and well-being.

Acknowledging this individual responsibility enhances rather than detracts from the sharing quality within a relationship, as there is no sense of obligation or pressure. The energy shared between two partners who are at peace within themselves and who trust each other makes that sense of well-being soar to new heights, as the individual strength of each partner feeds the other. And, of course, when one is temporarily down, the other can raise that energy up again.

If, on the other hand, we are talking about a relationship which is built on an image or a need, rather than the deep-rooted connection and flow between two trusting, open spirits, then that relationship will work on exactly the level of the projection. If you are only sharing a part of yourself, or if you allow your partner to share only part of him or herself because you see that partner as an image which does not reflect his or her true self, then the energy shared between you cannot be one of complete harmony and balance – and, ultimately, the cracks will appear.

So often, I have seen a relationship where one person leaves his or her partner for another person and the one left behind wallows in self-pity as the injured party. But do not let yourself be fooled by this; if the energy goes out of a relationship, it is because the connection is no longer or perhaps never has been deep down between the core of these two individuals. If you are honest with yourself, your intuition will always tell you the state of a relationship at any time; so many people intuitively feel a change within a relationship, but are afraid to confront it until it is too late. For we all change, and if you are open with your parnter and share these changes, then they do not have to lead you apart.

All of these examples above show how we have subconsciously *chosen* to relate to an individual in a certain way. The way we relate to people on a day to day basis – not just to that special partner, our family or close friends – demonstrates to what level our heart centre is truly open. If we find ourselves continuously judging other people or seeing them as extensions of ourselves, then we are still rooted in the centre of power. The true energy of love can only flow if we learn to recognize each individual as a complete being unto him- or herself.

In failing to understand the meaning of love and thereby failing to have that foundation of love in our lives, we impair the effectiveness of all the physical connections within the heart centre: the heart itself, the thymus and the immune system.

The essential question is: 'How deeply and truly do you want to relate?' The honest answer you give is a guide to what love really means to you.

Love: the Great Healer

A relationship can only blossom and grow if it is built on trust. Trust is the ability to open yourself up without reservations or conditions to another person and to see that person as he or she is. This is the basis of love in its clearest and purest sense.

I have just illustrated this in terms of a relationship with a 'special partner', but love works far beyond this limited sphere.

Love is a state of being, not a specific emotion. Remember this. If one lives with love as a state of being throughout one's existence, one will never be seriously sick, as the heart centre will remain open and the thymus and immune system will remain active and unimpared. If you are already sick, then this is the time to understand about love and bring it deep into your being.

Just think for a moment of people, such as Mother Teresa, who radiate nothing but love and you will begin to understand what love as a state of being means.

Let us start at the beginning again.

Love is concerned only with relating to people, including yourself. All else falls away as irrelevant.

Love has nothing to do with relating to people on a superficial level. You may be with someone as long as you like. You may talk to them, hug them, kiss them, have sex with them, but, unless you really open your heart to them, this has nothing to do with love.

Love starts with yourself. If you are unable to love yourself, you cannot know how to love others. If you are able to see yourself as you are and delight in yourself, then the light is beginning to shine within you.

If you deny yourself love, whether through guilt, fear, self-judgment or a general feeling of lack of worthiness, you are closing down your heart centre and the Healer Within. More fundamentally, you are denying yourself that essence within you from which emanates the joy and inner peace that you deserve in every aspect of your life.

Self-love is self-worth, the knowledge that you are worthy of the highest and best in your life and especially worthy of receiving love. If you open yourself to receive love from others, then the love you will give to yourself and to others will increase and increase. Likewise, if you open your heart to others, then you will receive in return, if you accept that you are worthy to do so.

This, in particular, is very important to understand. Love is the balance of giving and receiving and the breaking of that balance can allow AIDS to enter into your being. I have seen this occur where a person, who is a wonderful warm and loving being, giving of himself to all around him, cannot accept the love offered in return because of a deep down feeling, inspired within him many years back, that he is not worthy of receiving love.

Love just is. It is neutral. Love in its highest form is *perfect balance*. This is why it is the great healer, for in opening one's spirit, one allows the constant, harmonious flow of light to feed the heart and thymus, bringing health and energy to body and soul.

Love is not the wishy-washy emotion they sing about in love songs; it is a force like a burning arrow that cuts through all the dark and fuzzy aspects of your life. It means delving deep into yourself and into others. Love sees things clearly and truly as they are; if you are at peace with that loving part of yourself, you will see through the masks that others erect around themselves and you will see them as they are. You will see your own and others' true potential.

Love is forgiveness and releasing.

Love is freedom, as it has no ties.

Love is not just going through life being nice and sweet to people. Love and compassion are not to be confused with sympathy. Sympathy is where you enter into the spirit of someone's pain and thereby give it energy; compassion is feeling for someone in their pain, but standing apart from it and guiding that person out of it. Compassion can sometimes appear to be direct, cool and even cruel, but love itself is a cutting force sweeping away all superfluous emotional attachments.

Sympathy for oneself or self-pity, as it is better known, is not showing oneself love, as it is giving energy to one's pain. The healing force of self-love can only be felt if one stands back and rises out of pain and disease, nurturing the creative and loving part of oneself.

Love is trusting your instinct in relationships, knowing that, by showing your true self to the world, you will attract towards you those who are of the same energy as yourself, without even having to look for them. Then, there will be no emptiness, no isolation, as you will always have around you those with whom you can share, with whom not even words need be spoken to express the bond of love between you.

But, even more than this, love is an expression of our divine relationship with that almighty Whole, the Universe, which surrounds us wherever we are. It is an expression of the aspiration which we all have deep inside us to live always in peace, harmony and stillness with everything and everyone around us.

It is in that space of stillness that we listen to our inner voice and follow the path of our own individual creativity.

The Fifth Chakra: Communication and Expression

If love is the highest form of spirit on the earthly plane, then our expression of this and other aspects of our creativity can only bring the highest feeling of peace and fulfilment within us.

There are so many ways open to us to express our creativity and our highest selves; each one of them lifts us up away from the heavier, lower aspects of ourselves into that realm where we feel the freedom of being at one with ourselves and the world. We can express ourselves through words and touch, singing and dancing, smiling and laughing, to name but a few.

All these means of self-expression and communication are no less open to us when we feel down, for immediate expression of emotion, whether anger or sorrow or grief, is the only way to release it before it is allowed to fester and destroy the balance within. That is why tears are so important, as they are a natural, spontaneous release of sorrow, even sometimes an expression of joy.

In our second chakra, we learn to release our emotions, our sense of limitation and recognize our creativity. In the third, we learn to recognize our inner strength and, in the fourth, we feel the true meaning of love. But, all of this knowledge is worthless if we do not find an outlet for it, a means of expressing it and communicating it to others. The interrelationship which binds this Universe together depends on a continuous flow of communication, from the simple act of a bee pollinating a flower to the interchange of ideas and feelings between two people.

When life seems to be on a downward trend, it is so easy for one to retreat into one's shell. Sometimes, it is necessary to do so in the short term in order to settle into oneself and understand what is going on within; yet, making a habit of this leads to a melancholy within the soul and a gradual withdrawal from the natural energy which constant interchange brings into one's life.

If you are sick, it is all the more tempting to crawl into a dark hole, yet this is actually the time to do the opposite and begin to open yourself up not only to your inner self, but also to the world outside, to the friends who are trying to help you, to the new people in your life whom you meet and who share your predicament.

The challenge of overcoming disease is a true test of your creativity, and creativity cannot be expressed and fulfilled without communication. It is there to be shared and, even though responsibility rests with the individual, the energy between even just two people who share the same goal of banishing AIDS from their bodies and consciousness doubles the strength of the Healer Within each of them.

AIDS for many people presents the first opportunity to stand back from their lives and say: 'I am confronted with the possibility of dying. If I am really going to choose to live, what is it that I really want from this life ahead of me?' And the question itself is a release; it is an act of letting go of the need to hold on to all the superficial rubbish that has for so long drawn energy away from the essence of our lives.

What you are left with is the freedom to express your highest self, to do and to be all the things that you have deep down known to be important to you. It is the time to appreciate your own self-worth, to open your heart up to the world around you and to draw into your sphere and truly communicate with people who are of your nature. Most important of all, it is the time to follow your intuition and do exactly what you *feel* is right, without fear, or self-doubt.

The Power of Words

It is amazing how few people really understand the power of words. Words are at the heart of our creativity.

As long as a thought remains in your own mind, it is confined to yourself, your own personal sphere of reference. As soon as this thought is expressed in words, it is released from the confines of your own being and becomes universal.

That is why, even on a day to day basis, I always say: 'Be aware of what you speak.' Within the Universe, there is a natural balance and therefore whatever you put out from your own lips will create a certain reality which will return to you in one way or another. Just look closely at someone who is always finding fault in others and you will see how unharmonious that person's life will be on nearly every level.

We have the gift of communication and that is exactly what we have it for: to communicate. If you use communication for expressing negativity, you are not only wasting that gift, but you are creating an aura of negativity around you which will attract further negativity in your life. Each time you use words to complain about your lot, these words increase the power that this situation has over you. Likewise, if you are constantly 'bitching' about other people, you are giving them power over you and you will continue to attract negative people around you.

Communication is the means we have of relating to people, but it can also be abused to do the contrary. The spoken word can be used as a powerful tool for concealing what is really going on inside you, either through deceit or, more often, the habit of 'making' conversation on a level that has nothing to do with genuine communication.

That is why it is important to feel comfortable with silence. Many people, out of the habit of talking on a superficial level, feel uncomfortable when confronted with even a short period of silence in someone's company. Yet, when you are in the company of someone with whom you feel at ease, silence enables you to communicate on so many different levels – subliminal exchanges which Western man has lost because of his reliance on the spoken word.

As an extension of the way in which we relate to others, the way in which we communicate is a fundamental choice in our lives. If we choose to hide behind our words, we are choosing to suppress our true self with all the imbalance that such a decision brings; if we choose to communicate freely and express our inner selves, then our true nature flows freely outwards and, in joining with others, is reinforced.

The greatest strength of the spoken word is as an expression of faith, an affirmation that we can create our own reality. Through the spoken word, we can put out our innermost hopes and desires to connect with that limitless energy within the Universe.

I have already written about faith as the understanding of our link with this Universal Energy and our ability to bring this energy into our own being to create what we choose in our lives. It is through the word that we put this into action.

To give you an idea of the power of words, let us concentrate on two words which have great individual power: Yes and No. We have all seen how a powerful utterance of the word No can have a cowering effect on a dog, but have you ever seen it work in your own life? At any point in the next few days, if you see a situation coming towards you that you do not want to be part of you, just close your eyes, visualize this situation and shout either out loud or powerfully within yourself the word NO. When you do that, see how the word No creates an energy around it shattering anything in its path.

The word No is a particularly powerful tool in this instance if there is a fear that constantly keeps plaguing your mind. For instance, if you keep on getting an image inside your mind of you becoming sick, launch a NO towards it and see the effect it has. The very way the word is pronounced, in whatever language, has an energy that disrupts anything in its path.

Likewise, the sound of the word Yes has the quality that draws something towards you and it can be used for just that. If there is something which you truly desire and you know is right for you, yet there seem to be too many obstacles around it, then visualize it and put the energy of the word Yes out towards it and see how the obstacles crumble. First of all, you have to know what you truly want or do not want to be part of your life and then you put out the energy of Yes or No to it.

As I previously said, a thought remains in our private sphere until expressed. In verbalizing it, not only do we bring it out into the world, but the process of doing so forces us to transform what may have been a somewhat vague thought in our minds into something that we have to understand and express in a concrete manner. Writing one's thoughts down has a similar effect, which is why I often tell people to keep a journal during periods of profound change. Even writing this book has made me express ideas which were previously only vague concepts.

If you are reading this book, it is likely that you are undergoing a major period of change in your life, so I am going to ask you now to use the power of the spoken word.

MEDITATION NO. 9

In your own time, just sit in a quiet place and centre yourself. Then, focus on the past and specifically on all those aspects of your life which you do not wish to carry with you into the future. Hopefully, you have by now let go of most people and situations that have caused you pain, but here I wish you also to focus on all those traits in your behaviour which you do not like and which you feel limit your ability to create your own reality.

As you say out loud: 'I let go of . . . and do not want it to be part of my life again', you understand exactly what it is that you are releasing and you see that limitation pour out of your being.

You continue to do this until everything is exhausted and you can even write these things down as you identify them – the act of doing this often creates connections in your mind and makes you think of something else that lay hidden.

Once you are satisfied that you have covered all that needs to be covered, just let your mind go blank and focus on your present self.

Then, gradually allow to come to the surface the most important, the deepest aspirations and desires you have for the present and the future. One by one, see them within you and speak them out loud, affirming that they will happen. And each time an image of yourself in a creative guise comes to your mind, affirm this deepest part of you with the words: I AM.

Whatever it is that you are asking for which will point you towards your highest potential, you do it with the faith that, in putting it out to the Universe, the Universe will provide through its intricate, infinite connections. And if you have doubts about the effectiveness of such affirmations, then put it out there that you may learn faith and learn to accept that it is your God given right to have harmony, stillness, joy and love in your life.

The Sixth Chakra:
the Rational
and the Intuitive

Despite these doubts, deep down you feel that this natural balance and harmony in the world is right and can be drawn upon into your own life – it is your rational mind that has the doubt. Nothing that I write will be of any worth to you unless it feels right – and even the sense of it feeling right may be submerged by that rational part of you that needs tangible proof of everything before you accept it.

As I come to the end of the main part of this book, I am going to spend a little time explaining the essence of those two seemingly opposite sides of us: the rational and the intuitive. The way in which we allow one to dominate the other is probably the most fundamental imbalance within us, which filters down into all the other aspects of our behaviour – remember how I wrote about the pituitary and pineal glands at the beginning of the book and how they basically control all the other parts of the endocrine system below them.

From his early origins as a creature of instinct, man's rational faculties have grown at an ever increasing rate to reach their peak at the time we are in now. But, what exactly is this thing which we call the rational mind?

I prefer to call it the sequential mind as the key to its growth is sequence: as man sees and understands one part of his existence, this leads him to an understanding of the next stage. What the sequential mind is in fact doing is taking each part of the Whole which is the Universe and dividing it up into little parcels of knowledge which our limited faculties can grasp. In doing so, man started by first being able to understand individual parts of this whole, his environment, until this understanding of it gradually increased to the point where he can even harness and alter parts of it.

This is seeing the rational, sequential mind from a global standpoint. Of much more relevance to AIDS and health is the way in which the development of the rational mind affects us on a personal level, in particular with regard to the way we relate to the world around us.

From an early age, most of us are sent to school, following an education which is designed almost exclusively to develop our rational faculties. Whether in mathematics and science or history and economics, we are given specific pieces of information to learn and then to relate to each other. Our so-called intelligence is judged on our ability to absorb these countless bits of information, and, as we grow older, our 'usefulness' in the world is in turn judged by this 'intelligence'.

In dividing everything we do, see or experience into so many different and often seemingly unrelated little parcels, it is not surprising that our minds are never still or that you hear people so often say: 'Oh! I never seem to have time to sit down and relax.' This constant darting of the mind from one thing to another is probably the most common addiction of the urbanized Western world – an addiction it certainly is, as it is a means of giving up one's power by constantly worrying about and putting energy into a whole diversity of things that have no real, deep bearing on our lives. In addition, the impatience which arises from this state of mind never allows one to truly settle within that stillness, that giving and receiving state of being which I described as love earlier on.

As you might have imagined, this leads me back once more to that same old question of balance. If you are a person whose mind is never at rest and needs constantly to be occupied doing or worrying about something, you not only create tension and stress which affects the whole of your endocrine system. Of even more importance is the fact that you are constantly drawing energy out of yourself away from that true essence within you, denying that essential intuitive half of your mind and leaving emptiness in its place.

So, what is intuition?

In contrast to the rational mind, which divides everything into little pieces and must have explanations for everything, our intuitive mind is that part of us which sees and accepts the Whole. The rational mind is active, always doing; the intuitive mind is passive and receptive. The intuitive mind is what we call instinct, whereby we do things spontaneously without conscious thought. It is that part of us from where we get thoughts out of the blue and we wonder where they come from!

The most elemental example of the intuitive mind common to all living creatures is the survival instinct. As a species, man has always been a social animal, so the importance we place on relationships in our lives is also a fundamental instinct. Yet, what is most relevant to us here is the intuitive part of us which is particular to each one of us, which creates our own individuality.

Our individuality is of course partly created by the accumulation of experiences throughout our lives, but there is something more to it than that, a vague quality within each person which is distinguishable from any other person.

This is the intuitive part of an individual which resides in the sixth chakra, the third eye, and which rises up through the seventh, the crown chakra to connect with the Whole, the limitless energy and order of God, the Universe. As with those thoughts that come to us out of the blue, this connection is what makes us feel when things are right, as the information and thoughts we receive in this manner come from a source which sees the whole picture. Instead of the limited view of reality seen by our rational mind, our intuitive mind guides us in a direction, which goes far beyond the scope of our understanding, towards our highest potential – a potential which we may at this point in our lives not be able to comprehend. In the case of AIDS, a disease which at first sight seems to mean nothing but pain and suffering has the potential, if you follow the strength of your intuition, to open a whole new vision of life for you.

This is why faith and intuition are inextricably bound together – in trusting your intuition, you have faith that this is your connection to the Universe which will guide you to your highest good in all that you do.

And this in turn is why I always say to people, especially in these times: 'Always follow your intuition'. Every so often, something will come to your mind that just feels right: a feeling that you should embark on a new course in whatever aspect of your life, a feeling so strong that you cannot avoid making a decision.

The important thing is that, if you feel something strongly enough, you should do it. It is fairly inevitable that, along with this intuitive feeling, your rational mind will come up with lots of little objections, such as 'It's too risky', 'What will people think?' or 'My doctors would not approve'.

Well, the ultimate question is: do you wish to live the rest of your life in fear and through the eyes of others or do you wish to be yourself and follow that inner part of yourself? Just another choice!

It may appear that what I am doing here is exalting the intuitive over the rational mind, but this is not the case.

In our modern, 'civilized' world, the behaviour of most people is governed ninety per cent by the rational mind and ten per cent by the intuitive mind. What I am saying is that we should allow the intelligence of our rational understanding to be at one with our spiritual nature. We should learn to recognize when our intuition is tapping into the broader picture which our rational mind cannot see.

On a physiological level, this is what the right and left side of the brain are all about and it is the cerebral cortex which links the two so that they can work together. And (you must be getting rather bored of this word by now!), what about balance? Right at the beginning of this book, I wrote about the pineal and pituitary glands, which are the masters of the endocrine system. Quite simply, if there is balance within this sphere of our being, then balance and health will reign in the rest of our body.

So, you may ask, if balance between intuition and rationality will bring the rest of the body into balance, why bother with the rest of the book? The answer, and you will see as you look at your own behaviour, is that all these things we have been letting go of, from fear to guilt, jealousy to judgment, are all products of a rational mind devoid of intuitive input. They are all aspects of our lives which have been parcelled off and have been given a surplus of energy, taking away from the natural energy, flow and balance of the whole.

Throughout this book, I have been suggesting meditations which have all been fairly specific. This final one is what I call the 'Maintenance Meditation'. It is, by and large, what I do every day both in the morning and the evening, and, once you get used to it, it need only take ten minutes.

It may be that you already do your own regular meditation, which is fine. This is for people who wish to get started, but I always say that you must in the end follow whatever feels right for you.

The essence of meditation is to bring stillness into your life at the beginning and end of every day. If this book has at all changed your perception of life, or if changes are happening to you anyway, it is so important to make a point at least twice a day of calmly entering your own space and just being there within yourself.

To begin with, meditation can be a bit of a struggle, as your mind will keep hopping in lots of different directions. This does not matter. Just be aware of yourself doing this, let go of whatever distracting thought you have and return to that central part of yourself. Do not fight it. In the end, it will become second nature, and the freshness and lightness you will feel after just a few minutes of inner peace will be something you can draw upon at any time of the day.

In the summer and whenever I can, I will always do my meditation leaning against a tree trunk, as this really gives me a sense of connection with the earth, but the important thing is to choose a place which is as quiet as possible. I also find that sitting as erect as possible always helps – otherwise, I have a tendancy to doze off!

MEDITATION NO. 10

You begin this meditation by closing your eyes and then grounding and running your energies in exactly the way that I described in Meditation No. 1 at the beginning of the book. Once you are comfortable with this, instead of opening your eyes, you continue as follows.

What you are going to do first of all is to visualize your chakras. At first this may be a little difficult but, once you have a feel of them, it will come to you very easily. It may even be that visualizing them is not right for you – it may be better to sense their position in your body and feel the different currents of energy in these parts of your body.

In a visual sense, your chakras are like whirlpools or tornados of energy starting off at their widest point two inches away from the body and at the narrowest point attached to the spinal cord.

Your first chakra is attached to your coccyx bone at the base of your spine and faces downwards towards the earth. At its widest point, two inches from the body, it is about the width of a golf ball.

Your second chakra is situated two fingers' width below your navel. It is attached to the spinal cord at that level and faces outwards two inches in front of your body – at its widest point, it is about the width of a tennis ball.

Your third chakra is located in the solar plexus area just beneath the breastbone and is the same size as the second.

Your fourth chakra is at the level of your heart, although, unlike the heart itself, it is in that central part of you attached to your spinal cord. It is the same size as the second and third.

Your fifth is located in your throat and is about the size of the first.

Your sixth is in the central part of your forehead just above the eyebrows and is the same size, maybe a little smaller than the fifth.

Your seventh points upwards to the sky above you connecting to that central part of the brain, and, at its widest point two inches above the body, is about the size of the rim of a coffee mug.

You focus on these seven chakras and see or feel them all aligned in a straight line along your spinal cord.

Then, you concentrate on the three lower chakras and see a narrow, hollow cord stretch out from each of them all the way from the spine out into the distance.

Focusing in turn on the first, second and third, you see a brilliant gold light shooting towards your body from some point in the distance and this in turn enters each of your three lower chakras. As that bright light energy comes flowing into each chakra, it disturbs all the dark mass, like a thick layer of grime and dust, which has been allowed to accumulate there over the years – in the second, this black grime represents all the emotional charges that you have been hanging on to all these years and, in the third, it is all the imbalance of power and judgment etc. that you have allowed to build up inside you.

And, as this gold light breaks up this dark, lifeless energy inside you, it sweeps all the darkness out from inside you through the hollow cord attached to your chakra and out into the universe. So, as the light initially spreads into your chakra, the light that comes out through the cord is darkened by this layer upon layer of dirt being swept out with it. As the light continues to pour in and more and more heaviness is swept away, the light leaving through the cord gradually becomes brighter and brighter until it is just as bright as the gold light coming in. Then, all the dark energy has been swept away.

Once you have finished this to your satisfaction, you let the cords just slip away into the distance and see and feel each of those lower aspects of yourself filled with a new light energy.

Then, you focus on your upper four chakras and repeat the process. As the light flows into your heart chakra, you feel being expelled all those parts of you which say that you are not worthy of love and which prevent you from giving love out to others. As it becomes clearer, you feel the whole energy of your heart expand, not just from the light from outside, but also, now that it has been freed, that true essence of yourself which is and always will be within, flowing through every aspect of your being. When you finally allow the cords to disappear and the gold light fade, there comes from within an image of a beautiful pink rose which radiates its own loving energy throughout your being, filling your whole body with life and energy, stimulating your heart and immune system, radiating health in every cell and destroying any foreign body or virus which does not belong there.

When you are satisfied that your whole body is radiating with this energy of light, you move up to your throat centre and see the gold light pouring in, not only clearing out all those ties that prevent you expressing your true creativity, but also spreading down your arms to your fingertips filling them with the light and energy of creativity. And, as you have expelled all the darkness from this fifth chakra, you allow the cord and the gold light to fade away and, from within streams out a blue light, the ray of communication which is that natural expressive part of you.

You then move up to your third eye, and, as the gold light pours in, you see it expand, and as the light passes through the opening, it enters what seems like an enormous cavern stretching far beyond the imaginings of your own mind. This dark cavern becomes brighter and brighter, larger and larger as the light continues to flow in through your third eye, until there seem to be no walls to this cavern, only a ceiling. And, as you look above you, you see this ceiling burst open with a flash of light entering from above through your Crown Chakra, combining the limitless knowledge and energy of the Universe with that space, which is your own individuality. And you feel yourself standing in the middle of this limitless light and space around you, knowing that this is the energy which is there both within and outside you, the two fusing together, to be drawn into your being at will.

As you feel this energy, you see your body in your mind's eye and, as you breathe deeply, you see the light that is radiating within it expand one then two feet beyond the contours of your physical body. You allow that energy of light, your own space, to remain there knowing that it is there to protect you from any outside force which does not belong to your being.

So, for a while, you just sit there, allowing this freedom, this essential energy of light within you, to become familiar to you.

Then, finally you open your eyes and put your hands down on the ground to let any excess energy flow out into the earth.

4

AIDS – A Broader Perspective

I am sure most of you have heard the term: 'The New Age'. I am not so wild about such specific terms myself, but the truth is that we have entered into a period of change on this planet which has not occurred to this extent for thousands of years. I am not talking about material and technological change, although this is all part of it; I am referring to a fundamental shift in Consciousness.

The old age was the Age of Pisces and the figure who introduced this age in the West was Jesus Christ, Christ the Fisherman. He, like Buddha and others before him, was a prophet, teacher and healer of immense stature, and, if you strip down the dogma which has been added to his life and words since he left this planet, he taught two very basic things: 'God is Love' and 'God is Within You'.

His life and actions were, in a sense, a spark, a legacy laid down for us living in the world today. Following his death, the world became enmeshed in a vibration, where power, manipulation and control have ever since been the essential hallmarks of our behaviour, especially of the behaviour of our leaders.

The 'organized' religions of today have sadly led the way in this respect and have much to answer for, as they so imperiously set themselves up as the keepers of the spiritual side of man. From as early as the fourth century AD when the Roman Emperor Constantine espoused Christianity for political reasons, the hierarchy of the Christian Church has often been more interested in power than love. (Of course, Christianity has been the inspiration of some of the most blessed, influential figures in our history, but their inspiration came from an *individual* faith and sense of purpose.)

It is a constant source of amazement to me how organized religion continues to pour energy into negativity and hate rather than focus on good and love. For so many of my generation, religion means nothing because the spirit has been taken out of it. The Catholic Church spends all its energy on sin and guilt, the so-called 'Fundamentalists' preach a regime of intolerance and self-righteousness. This has nothing to do with Spirit; it has everything to do with power.

I have mentioned this perversion of Christ's teaching here, because this 'New Age' into which we have entered is basically a renewal of that spark which may be called the True Christ Consciousness, where each individual finds the God within him or herself.

To those of you for whom the words Christ and Christianity have bad or even absurd connotations, let me explain what I mean by the Christ Consciousness. The word Christ was a term used to describe the human being we know as Jesus, but is not inseparable from Jesus. It is a Consciousness – Jesus happened to be at that time in history the vehicle for spreading the teachings of this Consciousness. Therefore, the return of the Christ Consciousness has nothing to do with the man Jesus; it is the return of his very simple teachings which have been forgotten: 'God is Love' and 'God is Within'. In other words, it means that the Earth and Mankind, as the highest form of Consciousness on the Earth, will raise themselves out of the power vibration into the vibration of love, out of the third chakra into our rightful place of the fourth chakra, the centre of the heart.

So, what does all this mean in terms of us as individuals and what does it have to do with AIDS?

On the personal level, the beginning of a new age or cycle is always heralded in by an incredible surge of energy into people's lives and the planet as a whole – an energy which makes the impetus for change and inner transformation stronger and stronger.

This energy has been gradually increasing for quite a few

years, but in particular burst through in the middle of 1987, and will continue at this pace for quite a few years to come.

AIDS, over the years, has transformed the consciousness of thousands of people, myself included, whereby it has nudged us along a different path in our lives. By the time you read this book, that nudge will have become like a giant booster rocket behind you – as a 'channel' friend of mine so aptly described it to me recently, the change of energy we are going through is like taking out a 40 watt bulb and replacing it with a 200 watt bulb.

This is why the process of letting go is so important. This surge of energy which is sweeping through our lives at this moment is so powerful that, if we are light with no attachments and encumbrances, we shall be swept along with it to the extent that we cannot imagine how much our lives will have been transformed within even a few years from now – not only in terms of the potential within us, but also in terms of the ease and peace which will fill our lives. If, on the other hand, we still have excess baggage on us, we are in for a bumpy ride, knocking our heads continuously on the obstacles we create for ourselves.

That is why it is so important to get to the point of releasing all this superfluous crap in your lives and learning to distinguish that voice of true intuition from the voice of fear. The choice is so simple: in following your intuition, your life will speed on; in giving into doubt and fear, in holding on to the past, these changes will pass you by. It does not matter if you do not know where these changes will lead you; if you are patient and follow that intuitive part of you, it will be made perfectly clear in time.

With regard to AIDS, this is the difference between having and not having the disease. As I write this book, there are people I know who are gradually clearing their body of AIDS and will be in total remission within a year. They are being swept forwards and so many new things, parts of themselves they had never imagined, are opening up before them.

Sure, there has been a lot of suffering with AIDS, but, on a global scale, this has been just one of the means for certain individuals to focus their attention deep within themselves. AIDS has been a catalyst to prepare certain people for this change in energy and, even for those who have died, it has been a process of growth. Life does not just end with physical death on this earthly plane.

On a global scale, AIDS is symbolic of the changes, the birth pains that the Earth is going through. AIDS is a disease, a consciousness which is primarily rooted in the third chakra, the centre of power and strength. To rise out of it, we must leave power behind and open our hearts to love in its broadest sense. This is exactly what the Earth and Humanity must and, indeed, will do.

So many people have said to me: 'What is so special about us? Aren't we being a bit arrogant and unrealistic to believe that we are going to herald such a change in the world when life has been this way as long as history remembers?' My reply is always that this is something you can only answer for yourself. If you feel that you do have something to contribute to the world which will move this transformation forwards, then it is so. Only if you feel it within yourself can it be so.

The period of time we are entering into is literally *what we have all been waiting for*. It sounds a bit simplistic, doesn't it? But, there has been an incredible sense of anticipation building up for so long, often subconsciously, within so many people and these changes are the fruition of that feeling. I can hardly keep count of the people I meet on a day to day basis in the most unlikely circumstances who have had this feeling awaken inside them recently and only need someone to express it to, in order to share it. People are crawling out of the woodwork, understanding that a time for change in the way we behave towards each other has come: a time for Love. And, if you acknowledge and freely express that spiritual, loving side of your nature, you too will continuously be drawn to others who are undergoing the same changes.

Like a wounded animal trapped in a corner, the old way

will fight to preserve itself and, over the next five years at least, there will be incredible conflict, especially in the Middle East, to the degree that any talk of a loving world may seem absurdly unrealistic. But, it will be the death throes of the Old Age.

What is important is to just let this be and understand that it has nothing to do with you; to fight, to judge, to get involved in this distant conflict will only be to give it energy. The important thing is for us all to live our own lives according to our hearts and conscience and intuition; by residing within that core of inner strength and cutting through intolerance and hate within our own sphere of influence, we allow the light of that Consciousness of Love to emanate into the hearts of others, spreading and growing until there is no room in the world for the consciousness of power.

Again, if you feel that this is unrealistic, you have not taken in what this book is all about: responsibility. Not only do we have responsibility for our own lives; accepting that responsibility means that we are accepting responsibility for change within the world as a whole. If you say with a tone of defeat: 'What can I do to change the world?', you are denying that system of interrelationships, of eternal connections which makes up our Universe.

You have no doubt heard of the 'Domino' theory. Well, it does not have to refer to one country after the other falling under the 'spell of Communism'; it refers more relevantly to one individual changing another changing another changing another – ultimately changing the mass of humanity. And, of course, it is not just happening in your own back yard; this new awareness, this new consciousness is raising its head everywhere, quietly at first, but soon to have the force of a tidal wave.

And you know it!

One final word.

As you awaken to your own higher consciousness, it is a natural progression that you will be drawn to others and meet, seemingly by chance, people who are going through the same process.

You may feel that you need some guidance and you will find that there will be no shortage of teachers.

Remember two things. First of all: 'God is Within'. A teacher can only take you so far, and, in the end, you have to find your own way by listening to the voice within.

Secondly: choose your teacher carefully. If you feel you need one, follow your intuition as to who is right for you. Do not immediately accept one because someone you know has done so. This person may be a wonderful teacher, but the important thing is that he or she must be of your energy, must feel right for you.

And beware – (I hate to sound like a prophet of doom, but this is a necessary warning) – of false teachers. If you come across one who says that his or hers is the only way, or if you find that this person has allowed to build around him or her a circle of admirers, then stay clear. I have come across quite a few – they are still in the power vibration; they are not coming from the egoless state of Love.

So, I hope and trust that AIDS, as it has been for me, will be a wonderful vehicle for change in your life, so that you may rise out of the natural sense of fear that the word inspires and enter into a new world of your own inner strength, love and, of course, peace, happiness and laughter.

If you have anything you wish to write to me about which seems unclear, please do not hesitate to do so, c/o Amethyst Books, and I shall write back as soon as I can.